Sexual Dysfunction in Women

About the Author

Marta Meana, PhD, is a renowned sex researcher and therapist whose work on female sexuality has been widely published in the academic literature and extensively covered in national and international popular media. Professor of psychology at the University of Nevada, Las Vegas, she is president of the Society for Sex Therapy and Research, associate editor of the *Archives of Sexual Behavior*, and an advisor to the DSM-5 Workgroup on Sexual and Gender Identity Disorders.

Companion volume in this series:

David L. Rowland (2012)
Sexual Dysfunction in Men
ISBN 978-0-88937-402-7

Advances in Psychotherapy – Evidence-Based Practice

Series Editor
Danny Wedding, PhD, MPH, Professor of Psychology, California School of Professional
   Psychology / Alliant International University, San Francisco, CA

Associate Editors
Larry Beutler, PhD, Professor, Palo Alto University / Pacific Graduate School of Psychology,
   Palo Alto, CA
Kenneth E. Freedland, PhD, Professor of Psychiatry and Psychology, Washington University
   School of Medicine, St. Louis, MO
Linda C. Sobell, PhD, ABPP, Professor, Center for Psychological Studies, Nova Southeastern
   University, Ft. Lauderdale, FL
David A. Wolfe, PhD, RBC Chair in Children's Mental Health, Centre for Addiction and Mental
   Health, University of Toronto, ON

The basic objective of this series is to provide therapists with practical, evidence-based treatment guidance for the most common disorders seen in clinical practice – and to do so in a "reader-friendly" manner. Each book in the series is both a compact "how-to" reference on a particular disorder for use by professional clinicians in their daily work, as well as an ideal educational resource for students and for practice-oriented continuing education.

The most important feature of the books is that they are practical and "reader-friendly:" All are structured similarly and all provide a compact and easy-to-follow guide to all aspects that are relevant in real-life practice. Tables, boxed clinical "pearls," marginal notes, and summary boxes assist orientation, while checklists provide tools for use in daily practice.

Sexual Dysfunction in Women

Marta Meana
Department of Psychology, University of Nevada, Las Vegas, NV

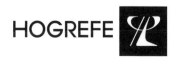

Library of Congress Cataloging in Publication

is available via the Library of Congress Marc Database under the
Library of Congress Control Number 2012935214

Library and Archives Canada Cataloguing in Publication

Meana, Marta, 1957-
    Sexual dysfunction in women / Marta Meana.

(Advances in psychotherapy--evidence-based practice ; 25)
Includes bibliographical references.
ISBN 978-0-88937-400-3

    1. Sexual disorders. 2. Psychosexual disorders. 3. Sexual
disorders--Treatment. 4. Psychosexual disorders--Treatment.
I. Title. II. Series: Advances in psychotherapy--evidence-based
practice ; 25

RC556.M43 2012   616.6'9   C2012-901850-3

PUBLISHING OFFICES
USA: Hogrefe Publishing, 875 Massachusetts Avenue, 7th Floor, Cambridge, MA 02139
               Phone (866) 823-4726, Fax (617) 354-6875; E-mail customerservice@hogrefe-publishing.com
EUROPE: Hogrefe Publishing, Merkelstr. 3, 37085 Göttingen, Germany
               Phone +49 551 99950-0, Fax +49 551 99950-425, E-mail publishing@hogrefe.com

SALES & DISTRIBUTION
USA: Hogrefe Publishing, Customer Services Department,
               30 Amberwood Parkway, Ashland, OH 44805
               Phone (800) 228-3749, Fax (419) 281-6883, E-mail customerservice@hogrefe.com
EUROPE: Hogrefe Publishing, Merkelstr. 3, 37085 Göttingen, Germany
               Phone +49 551 99950-0, Fax +49 551 99950-425, E-mail publishing@hogrefe.com

OTHER OFFICES
CANADA: Hogrefe Publishing, 660 Eglinton Ave. East, Suite 119-514, Toronto, Ontario, M4G 2K2
SWITZERLAND: Hogrefe Publishing, Länggass-Strasse 76, CH-3000 Bern 9

Hogrefe Publishing
Incorporated and registered in the Commonwealth of Massachusetts, USA, and in Göttingen, Lower Saxony,
Germany

Printed and bound in the USA
ISBN: 978-0-88937-400-3

Preface

Nearly everyone will experience sexual difficulties at some point in the course of their lives. For many, these difficulties will at times rise to the level of a sexual dysfunction, as currently defined by the latest edition of the American Psychiatric Association's *Diagnostic and Statistical Manual of Mental Disorders,* 4th Edition, Text Revision (DSM-IV-TR; APA, 2000). This may be especially true for women. They consistently report less desire, arousal, and orgasm frequency than men, as well as more pain associated with penetration. Sexual dysfunctions are possibly the most prevalent of any of the disorders in the DSM. Their apparent ubiquity thus raises two important questions: (1) Might our definitions of sexual dysfunction be overinclusive and consequently serve to pathologize what are in fact typical sexual variations – a normal diversity of experience? (2) Why do most clinical psychologists feel less well equipped to treat sexual dysfunction than they do major depression or anxiety disorders, which are nowhere near as prevalent?

The first question is currently being hotly debated in the literature and in ongoing attempts to modify diagnostic criteria for female sexual dysfunctions in the next edition of the DSM (more on this to follow). The debate is fueled by concerns that current definitions of female sexual dysfunction have been derived from a male sexuality analog that assumes sex to be a pure drive (like hunger), divorced from its complex psychological, relational, and social contexts. The debate is really about the accurate definition of sexual function for women. Although the discussion may at times seem academic, it has important implications for clients and for their therapists, as both try to align expectations with reality while allowing for the wide diversity of sexual experience that exists.

In regard to the second question, most clinical psychologists feel inadequate in the treatment of sexual dysfunction primarily because they lack training. Although there are psychologists who specialize in anxiety and depression, it is expected that every graduate from a clinical psychology program in North America will be competent in the treatment of these disorders. Unfortunately, that is not the case for sexual dysfunction, despite its prevalence. A discussion of why this is so is beyond the scope of this book, but attempting to redress the lack of training is at its heart. Clinical psychologists can most definitely help their clients navigate and address sexual problems effectively. Sex therapy, after all, is based on many of the same theories, principles, and techniques that guide many other interventions (Binik & Meana, 2009).

I want to thank Dr. Danny Wedding, as well as Robert Dimbleby of Hogrefe Publishing, for inviting me to participate in this series and to bring the treatment of female sexual dysfunction into the general fold of our discipline. Too many women are suffering from sexual difficulties for us to restrict their care. I am indebted to the University of Nevada, Las Vegas, for the sabbatical leave that facilitated the writing of this book and to Sarah Jones and Taylor Oliver for their research assistance. Importantly, I also want to thank Tim, Candy, Camilla, and Miko – my circle of love.

Marta Meana, PhD
Las Vegas, NV

Dedication

A mi padre, Antonio Meana.

Table of Contents

1

Description

1.1   Terminology

There are six sexual dysfunctions in the *Diagnostic and Statistical Manual of Mental Disorders,* 4th Edition, Text Revision (DSM-IV-TR; American Psychiatric Association [APA], 2000) that apply or are specific to women's sexual response: hypoactive sexual desire disorder (HSDD; 302.71), sexual aversion disorder (SAD; 302.79), female sexual arousal disorder (FSAD; 302.72), female orgasmic disorder (FOD; 302.73) (sometimes referred to as anorgasmia), dyspareunia (not due to a medical condition) (302.76), and vaginismus (not due to a medical condition) (306.51). There have been few changes in terminology from the publication of the revised third edition of the DSM, although current proposals for changes to the DSM-5 (expected publication date in 2013) promise significant alterations to current diagnostic categories. The terminology in the *International Statistical Classification of Diseases and Related Health Problems,* 10th Edition (ICD-10; World Health Organization, 1992) is semantically similar to that in the DSM-IV-TR, with the exception of the inclusion in the ICD-10 of a sexual dysfunction (excessive sexual drive) currently being considered as an appendix addition to the DSM-5. See Table 1 for a comparison of terminology across diagnostic manuals.

The six female sexual dysfunctions in the DSM-IV may be collapsed into three for the upcoming DSM-5

Table 1
Comparison of Terminology Across Diagnostic Manuals for Sexual Dysfunctions in Women

DSM-III-R	DSM-IV-TR	ICD-10 (codes)	DSM-5 Proposed (as of April 1, 2012)
Sexual Desire Disorders			
HSDD	HSDD (302.71)	Lack or loss of sexual desire (F52.0)	*Sexual interest/ arousal disorder in women*
SAD	SAD (302.79)	Sexual aversion and lack of sexual enjoyment (F52.1)	*Possible removal*

Table 1 continued

DSM-III-R	DSM-IV-TR	ICD-10 (codes)	DSM-5 Proposed (as of April 1, 2012)
Sexual Arousal Disorders			
FSAD	FSAD (302.72)	Failure of genital response (F52.2)	*Sexual interest/ arousal disorder in women*
Orgasm Disorders			
Inhibited female orgasm	FOD (302.73)	Orgasmic dysfunction (F52.3)	*FOD*
Sexual Pain Disorders			
Dyspareunia	Dyspareunia (N/GMC)	Nonorganic dyspareunia (F52.6)	*Genito-pelvic pain/ penetration disorder*
Vaginismus	Vaginismus (N/GMC)	Nonorganic vaginismus (F52.5)	*Genito-pelvic pain/ penetration disorder*

Note. DSM-III-R = *Diagnostic and Statistical Manual of Mental Disorders,* 3rd Edition (APA, 1987); DSM-IV-TR = *Diagnostic and Statistical Manual of Mental Disorders,* 4th Edition, Text revision (APA, 2000); FOD = female orgasmic disorder; FSAD = female sexual arousal disorder; HSDD = hypoactive sexual desire disorder; ICD-10 = *International Statistical Classification of Diseases and Related Health Problems,* 10th Edition (World Health Organization, 1992); N/GMC = not due to a general medical condition; SAD = sexual aversion disorder.

1.2   Definition

To understand both existing and proposed criteria for the sexual dysfunctions in women, it is necessary to briefly review the model of the sexual response that has had the most influence on our definitions of dysfunction. A simultaneously physical and psychological experience, the sexual response engages both the brain and the body. From genital engorgement to lubrication to autonomic arousal to cognitive and emotional processes to relational ones, the sexual response is indeed a full body/mind experience. Partnered sex doubles the complexity as two body/mind experiences meet and influence each other.

1.2.1   Traditional Models of the Sexual Response

Masters and Johnson

The sexual response is simultaneously a psychological and physiological experience

Despite the acknowledged complexity of the sexual response, definitions of dysfunction have been most influenced by the model introduced by Masters and Johnson (1970), whose research focused on the autonomic and genital aspects of sexuality. They proposed that the sexual response basically progressed through four distinct and sequential phases: excitement, plateau, orgasm, and resolution. The excitement phase in women was described as consisting of:

- genital and clitoral engorgement,
- vaginal lubrication,
- swelling of the breasts and nipple erection, and
- increases in autonomic arousal, including heart rate and blood pressure.

The plateau phase was described as a period of maximum arousal just prior to orgasm, wherein the outer third of the vagina becomes hypertonic while the inner part expands. In addition, the uterus moves up in the pelvic cavity, and the clitoral glans retreats under its hood. The orgasm phase consists of spasmodic contractions of the pelvic floor muscles, at which time autonomic arousal peaks and is generally accompanied by an intense subjective feeling of pleasure. The resolution phase was basically described as the period during which the process of vasocongestion and autonomic arousal reversed itself.

Kaplan and Lief

The Masters and Johnson model was physiologically focused and linear. The sexual response started at one phase and progressed sequentially through to its end. Missing from the model, however, was a motivational state that would lead one to seek stimuli that would initiate the sexual response or to be responsive to said stimuli if they presented themselves. That motivational state, which we commonly refer to as sexual desire, was independently proposed by Kaplan (1977) and Lief (1977) as an integral first phase of the sexual response. The resulting triphasic model consisted of desire, excitement (subsuming Masters and Johnson's plateau phase), and orgasm. The new model of the sexual response retained the linear structure of the original one.

Having defined the "normal" sexual response, the aforementioned models provided the frame for the definitions of sexual dysfunction in the various editions of the DSM to date. Things could go awry at any one of three phases of the sexual response. A woman could have or develop problems of desire (HSDD or SAD), or problems relating to arousal (FSAD), or problems relating to orgasm (FOD). Pain with sex was a dysfunction that stood apart from these phases, although desire and arousal problems were often blamed, with little empirical support, for the existence of dyspareunia and vaginismus. More likely, as we shall see, it is pain with sex that leads to problems in all phases of the sexual response.

1.2.2 Challenges to Traditional Models of the Sexual Response

Since the publication of the DSM-IV in 1994, theorizing and research on women's sexuality has increased significantly. The results of these efforts have raised doubts about the extent to which the models of the sexual response that have shaped DSM diagnostic criteria accurately represent the sexual experience of women. In question are the implicit assumptions that (1) sexual desire is a spontaneous drive, (2) the sexual response is necessarily linear in its progression, (3) desire and arousal are separate constructs, and (4) psychological, relational, and social contexts and motivations are secondary to the physiologi-

Traditional models of the sexual response may not adequately depict the diverse experience of women

cal aspects of the sexual response. An accumulating body of evidence suggests that these assumptions may represent an inaccurate depiction of female sexuality. New models of the sexual response are being proposed to integrate empirical findings that suggest a more complex process.

Incentive-Motivation Model

A group of Dutch researchers have proposed an incentive-motivation model of the sexual response that veers away from desire as a spontaneous, internally generated drive (e.g., Both, Spiering, Everaerd, & Laan, 2004). They maintain that sexual motivation emerges in response to sexual stimuli which are then processed (sometimes below the level of consciousness) and give rise to sexual action. Sexual desire occurs when the physiological changes associated with arousal are consciously perceived by the individual. Note that in this model, arousal precedes desire, although the two might be difficult, if not impossible, to distinguish. Desire is considered the conscious/cognitive experience that propels sexual action once arousal has been detected. In addition, this model proposes that individuals differ in their propensity to be aroused or motivated toward sexual action, and that this propensity may be contingent on psychological, neuropsychological, and cultural factors. The incentive-motivation model has posed an impressive empirically supported challenge to the sequence proposed by traditional models of the sexual response. Desire may not, after all, precede arousal. Desire may sometimes be a response rather than an originating, spontaneous drive.

Basson's Model

In support of the ideas inherent in the incentive-motivation model, Basson (2007) has provided a circular model of the sexual response, applicable to both men and women, although it originated in response to the failure of traditional models to account for the experience of a significant number of women. In a series of expert opinion papers, she argued the following:

In some women, desire may be experienced as responsive rather than spontaneous with relational factors playing a substantial role

- A significant number of women do not report spontaneous desire, although they respond positively to sexual stimuli and feel desire primarily in response to such stimuli.
- The motivation for sex may often be nonsexual (e.g., emotional intimacy) but nonetheless result in arousal and desire.
- Competent sexual stimuli produce sexual arousal which, in turn, produces sexual desire (the motivation to get more of what feels good).
- What feels good encompasses more than mere sexual release. Pleasure also emanates from many associated rewards, such as feelings of closeness, intimacy, and love.

Some of these contentions and clinical observations have been supported by literature indicating that it is empirically difficult to tease apart sexual desire from sexual arousal. Women themselves are not able to reliably distinguish between the two (Brotto, Heiman, & Tolman, 2009; Graham, Sanders, Milhausen, & McBride, 2004). Finally, thrown into the mix is a literature that urges the field to consider the complex nonphysiological context in which sex takes places, including social and economic forces impinging on the freedom and expression of women (Tiefer, 2001). Within the past decade, the Masters and Johnson / Kaplan/Lief model started to look simplistic. Basson's model of the sexual response suggested multiple motivational starting points and fluid subsequent phases, the order of which varied when and if you could actually tease them apart.

The jury is out on which of these two sets of models best accounts for women's sexual responses (for reviews, see Hayes, 2011; Meana, 2010). The conclusion most likely to emerge is that there is a diversity of sexual responses. The linear model may be more representative of some women, while the circular model may be more representative of others. It is also likely that there are life-span and situational differences. Seemingly spontaneous, uncomplicated desire and arousal may be more common at younger ages, in newer relationships, or during periods of low stress. The more responsive, more situation-contingent version of sexual responding may be more representative of women as they age, during challenging life periods, or in long-term relationships. Regardless, the research of the last few years has clearly illustrated what most clinicians already knew impressionistically – that sexuality is complex and exists within a system that extends far beyond genital plumbing.

1.2.3   Sexual Dysfunctions in Women

Challenges notwithstanding, the Masters and Johnson/Kaplan/Lief model of sexual function remains the backdrop against which the DSM-IV sexual dysfunction criteria were devised. Recent research and the incentive-motivation and Basson models provide the frame for proposed revisions in the coming edition (DSM-5). The following section will consequently describe both current definitions and criteria, as well as summarize the latest recommendations for new ones. The best starting point is the criteria shared by all dysfunctions not attributed to general medical conditions, substance use, or medications.

All of the sexual dysfunctions have three diagnostic criteria (A, B, and C). Criterion A details the characteristics of each dysfunction. Criterion B ("The disturbance causes marked distress or interpersonal difficulty") is identical in all of them. This criterion stipulates that if the sexual presentation does not sufficiently concern the individual or cause any relationship problems, it is not diagnosable as a sexual dysfunction. This is a controversial criterion. Some think it is important to maintain it so that we do not pathologize individuals who are satisfied with their level of sexual function, whatever that may be (Meana, 2010). Others emphasize that no such concerns have overridden the diagnosis of other disorders in the DSM, for obvious reasons (e.g., a happy person with schizophrenia still has schizophrenia); a woman who has no orgasms still has orgasmic disorder whether she cares about it or not (Althof, 2001). Critics of the distress criterion have suggested that it become a specifier (i.e., an addendum that further describes the situation rather than determines the existence of a disorder). Current drafts of proposals for the DSM-5 appear to be maintaining the distress criterion despite objections.

Criterion C varies only slightly across dysfunctions and stipulates that the dysfunction cannot be better accounted for by (1) another Axis I disorder (except another sexual dysfunction), (2) the direct physiological effects of a substance (e.g., a drug of abuse, medication), and/or (3) a general medical condition. Exceptions occur in the case of SAD and the two sexual pain disorders. In the case of SAD, neither substances/medications nor general medical conditions are invoked as possible causes of the disorder. In the case of dyspareunia, the existence of vaginismus or lack of lubrication overrides the primary diagnosis of dyspareunia. In the case of vaginismus, substances/medications are not mentioned as possible culprits. Dysfunctions at any stage of the sexual response cycle that are attributed primarily to a general medical condition or to substance use or medication use have separate codes in the DSM-IV and will not be covered in this text.

All sexual dysfunctions in the DSM-IV-TR also have three dichotomous specifiers. The first (lifelong type / acquired type) relates to the onset of the disorder. The second (generalized type / situational type) refers in a basic way to contextual factors: Does the difficulty present itself in all situations, or is it limited to specific ones? The third specifier addresses etiology (due to psychological factors / due to combined factors). This last specifier is the most problematic as it asserts the possibility of disengaging physical from psychological factors in the sexual response. Arguably, such disengagement is neither within the reach of our current knowledge nor particularly realistic, considering that the sexual response is simultaneously physical and psychological.

Table 2
Criterion A for Each of the Sexual Dysfunctions Applicable to Women in DSM-IV-TR

Dysfunction	Monosymptomatic Criterion A
HSDD	Persistently or recurrently deficient (or absent) sexual fantasies and desire for sexual activity. The judgment of deficiency is made by the clinician, taking into account factors that affect sexual functioning, such as age and the context of the person's life.
SAD	Persistent or recurrent extreme aversion to, and avoidance of, all (or almost all) genital sexual contact with a sexual partner.
FSAD	Persistent or recurrent inability to attain, or to maintain until completion of the sexual activity, an adequate lubrication-swelling response of sexual excitement.
FOD	Persistent or recurrent delay in, or absence of, orgasm following a normal sexual excitement phase. Women exhibit wide variability in the type or intensity of stimulation that riggers orgasm. The diagnosis of FOD should be based on the clinician's judgment that the woman's capacity is less than would be reasonable for her age, sexual experience, and the adequacy of sexual stimulation she receives.
Dyspareunia	Recurrent or persistent genital pain association with sexual intercourse.
Vaginismus	Recurrent or persistent involuntary spasm of the musculature of the outer third of the vagina that interferes with sexual intercourse.

Note. DSM-IV-TR = *Diagnostic and Statistical Manual of Mental Disorders,* 4th Edition, Text revision (APA, 2000); FOD = female orgasmic disorder; FSAD = female sexual arousal disorder; HSDD = hypoactive sexual desire disorder; SAD = sexual aversion disorder.

The next three sections will describe each of the six female sexual dysfunctions, with a focus on Criterion A, which consists of the monosymptomatic defining characteristic of each disorder (Table 2).

Sexual Desire and Arousal Disorders

With regard to, or applicable to, women, the DSM-IV-TR lists two sexual dysfunctions related to purported impairments in sexual desire (hypoactive sexual desire disorder [HSDD] and sexual aversion disorder [SAD]) and one related to impairments in arousal (female sexual arousal disorder [FSAD]). The desire disorders are not defined in a gender-differentiated way, while, clearly, FSAD relates to aspects of female sexual arousal exclusively.

HSDD is defined as a persistent or recurrent deficiency or absence of sexual fantasies and desire for sexual activity. The judgment of deficiency or absence is left to the clinician, and the DSM specifies that this judgment be made in the context of potentially relevant factors, such as the person's age and the circumstances of their life. Although fantasies feature prominently in the definition of HSDD, most women who present with this problem are not concerned about their fantasy life. They are typically in relationships, and they present with distress about a level of desire that is disturbing to them and/or to their partners.

There are a number of ways HSDD can present, including:

(1) the single woman who has never had much sexual desire and is distressed by the fact that the world seems to revolve around something that barely registers for her (rare);

(2) the partnered woman who never had much desire for sex and was unconcerned about it until it started to interfere with a valued relationship (more common);

(3) the partnered woman whose level of sexual desire has decreased to an extent that is distressing to her and usually to her partner (quite common);

(4) the woman who would not be personally distressed by her level of desire were it not for the dissatisfaction and distress of her partner (quite common).

The distress can range from a wistful longing for an old feeling that appears to have faded, to symptoms of depression centered on the loss or decrease of desire. The interpersonal difficulty can range from a vague frustration about lack or loss of intimacy, to serious relationship-threatening discord over sexual frequency.

It is important to emphasize that HSDD is not diagnosed in relation to norms of sexual desire. There are no reliable norms regarding how often most women feel desire, and even if there were, they would not be particularly useful. Without distress or interpersonal difficulty, women would have no reason to seek help. If a woman does not want something and no one else wants her to want it, one could argue that there is no problem, even if the distress/interpersonal criterion is ignored. However, women do seek help because they are unhappy with their desire levels and/or because their partners are dissatisfied with the frequency of sex in the relationship. In concert with a voluminous research indicating a large difference in sexual desire/drive between men and women (Baumeister, Catanese, & Vohs, 2001), desire discrepancies feature prominently in clinical cases. This makes the diagnosis of HSDD in women tricky because (1) the partner's level of desire may be unduly influential in the assessment of the woman's supposed problem, and (2) by definition, the diagnosis pathologizes the partner with less desire, who, in heterosexual relationships, is more often than not the woman.

Deciding what is deficient sexual desire is a relative endeavor, as it is often measured against social expectations or a partner's desire

SAD is defined as persistent or recurrent extreme aversion or avoidance of all or most sexual activity with a sexual partner. Women with SAD generally present with feelings of revulsion regarding sex. The disgust is sometimes centered on a specific aspect of sex, such as genital secretions, but it is more often generalized to multiple, if not all, aspects of the sexual experience. Exposure to sexual stimuli or the prospect of sexual activity is aversive and can be accompanied with anxiety, fear, and anger at the perceived pressure to engage in acts that they find revolting.

The intensity of the aversion can range from mild anxiety and/or lack of pleasure to panic attack symptoms, including heart palpitations, shallow breathing, nausea, and dizziness. In most cases, the avoidance of sex is quite severe as these women will go to great lengths to avoid sex with their partners. Partners also report that when they do have sex, the disgust is usually quite apparent in facial expressions (e.g., wincing) and bodily movements (e.g., cringing). Consequently, the most common presentation of SAD is at the behest of a partner or out of the woman's concern for a relationship suffering under the stress of her aversion to sex.

The DSM-IV's inclusion of SAD under the sexual desire disorders clearly indicates the theory that SAD represents a deficit in desire. However, its clinical presentation is quite different from HSDD. There is clearly no sexual desire, but the distress generally relates to the perceived pressure to have sex rather than to the unfulfilled wish that desire would be present or return. In therapy, women with SAD can be quite expressive about their disgust and very anxious about treatment that will necessitate some hierarchy of exposure to sexual stimuli, no matter how finely graded the hierarchy. In contrast, women with HSDD are more likely to welcome ideas/exercises that might have a positive impact on their desire. As such, emotions, cognitions, and behavior that accompany SAD often appear to have much in common with Specific Phobia. On the other hand, mild levels of disgust and behavioral avoidance are also present in some women with HSDD (Sims & Meana, 2010). The question is thus whether SAD exists on the extreme negative end of a continuum of sexual desire or whether it represents a categorically different disorder governed by a different set of factors. In other words, is it more of an anxiety disorder or a sexual dysfunction?

Most women do not make much of a distinction between desire and arousal

FSAD is defined as a persistent or recurrent inability to attain or maintain an adequate level of vasocongestion and lubrication until the completion of sexual activity. This is clearly the sexual dysfunction that relates directly to the "excitement" phase of the sexual response, with excitement being defined exclusively in terms of changes related to arousal in the genitals. The literature, however, does not show much support for the existence of this dysfunction. It is reportedly rare for women to present with FSAD only, or with FSAD as their chief complaint (Graham, 2010a). There are a number of reasons this might be the case: (1) the high comorbidity between FSAD and other sexual dysfunctions, (2) lack of differentiation between desire and arousal, and (3) low levels of distress associated with impairments in physical indicators of arousal. Barring medical conditions or vaginal changes associated with age and menopause, women do not often report problems with physical arousal separate from problems with desire or orgasm or pain.

Sexual interest/arousal disorder in women is the new diagnostic category currently proposed for the coming edition of the DSM (DSM-5) (American Psychiatric Association, 2012). This category would subsume the current diagnoses of HSDD and FSAD with the rationale that (1) neither the empirical literature nor women themselves reliably distinguish desire from arousal, and (2) the high degree of comorbidity between the two diagnoses makes their separation questionable. In its preliminary draft, this proposed diagnostic category consists of a polythetic Criterion A requiring at least three out of five indicators of lack of sexual interest/arousal (absent or reduced interest in sexual activity, erotic thoughts/fantasies, initiation/receptivity, excitement/pleasure, genital/nongenital sensations) that have persisted for at least 6 months. Criterion B maintains distress or impairment. In addition to typifying whether the dysfunction is of the lifelong or acquired type, there is also a proposed list of six specifiers intended to reflect the various contextual and medical factors that can be implicated in any one woman's difficulty (generalized/situational, partner factors, relationship factors, individual vulnerability factors, cultural/religious factors, medical factors).

This new proposed diagnostic category recommended by the DSM-5 Workgroup on Sexual and Gender Identity Disorders will be subjected to further review and expert feedback, which may result in significant changes to this draft. The Workgroup has also recommended that SAD be removed as a distinct sexual dysfunction given its greater similarity to specific phobia.

Orgasm Disorder

Female orgasmic disorder (FOD) is defined as persistent or recurrent delay or absence of orgasm following a normal arousal phase. The DSM definition acknowledges that there is a wide variability in the type and intensity of stimulation that triggers orgasm and, as such, leaves it up to the clinician to determine if the woman's orgasmic capacity is less than might be expected for her age, sexual experience, and the competence of the stimulation she receives.

One would think that FOD would be relatively easy to diagnose since, unlike desire and arousal, it purportedly pertains to a discrete event. However, this is not necessarily the case. Unlike men, who usually ejaculate with orgasm, no such discrete event occurs with orgasm in women. Attempts to define orgasm have thus relied on extremely varied subjective descriptions (Mah & Binik, 2001), and a significant number of women are unsure whether or not they have experienced an orgasm (Meston, Hull, Levin, & Sipski, 2004). The other complicating factor in defining FOD relates to the competence of the stimulation the woman is receiving.

Despite decades of data indicating that the majority of women require clitoral stimulation to reach orgasm, there is a persistent expectation in the public that women should be having orgasm through intercourse. It is thus not unusual for couples to present in therapy with concerns about the woman's orgasmic capacity because she fails to reach orgasm through penetration alone. Another factor that makes the diagnosis of FOD far from obvious is the

A majority of women do not reach orgasm from the stimulation provided by intercourse alone

fact that, in contrast to men, there is great variability in the extent to which women find orgasm an important component of their sexual experience and satisfaction.

The DSM-5 Workgroup on Sexual and Gender Identity Disorders recommends that the diagnosis of FOD be maintained but that it be elaborated to include reduced intensity of orgasmic sensations and to account for the expected high comorbidity with sexual interest/arousal disorders as well as the varied contextual factors (the aforementioned six specifiers) that could be affecting the experience of orgasm (American Psychiatric Association, 2012).

Sexual Pain Disorders

The DSM-IV-TR lists two sexual pain disorders. One is applicable to both men and women: dyspareunia (not due to a general medical condition). The other is specific to women: vaginismus (not due to a general medical condition).

Dyspareunia is described simply as recurrent or persistent genital pain associated with sexual intercourse. The pain cannot be caused exclusively by vaginismus or lack of lubrication. Pain associated with sexual intercourse occurs primarily during penetration, but in some women, it can last for hours and even days after the sexual encounter. Although this pain had traditionally been linked etiologically with sexual activity, the genital pain of dyspareunia is also experienced with other types of penetration or stimulation to the genital area (e.g., tampon insertion, finger insertion, gynecological examinations, and varied other types of genital contact) (Meana, Binik, Khalife, & Cohen, 1997a).

Most women with dyspareunia have a pain condition that interferes with intercourse rather than a sexual problem resulting in pain

In fact, research indicates that the pain–sex link might be incidental in the majority of cases (Binik, 2010a). Pain is experienced during sex not because of any psychosexual or relational conflict, but rather because sex involves the mechanical stimulation of a hyperalgesic area. The penis, speculum, and tampon are all simply pain stimuli making contact with tissue that has become hypersensitive.

The clinical presentation of dyspareunia is typically quite clear. Women generally report a significant amount of distress about the fact that they find intercourse anywhere from moderately painful to excruciating. However, the question of how to rule out – or even whether we should rule out – a general medical condition is not clear at all. There are a number of conditions of unknown etiology (provoked vestibulodynia [PVD] being the most prominent) that probably account for the majority of cases of dyspareunia in premenopausal women. PVD is characterized by a severe, burning/sharp pain that occurs in response to pressure localized in the vulvar vestibule, which is essentially the entry point to the vagina. Conditions such as these often go unrecognized because the only obvious symptom to the untrained professional is pain with intercourse. Consequently, it is easy to psychologize or sexualize the symptoms, despite the fact that there are very few accounts in the empirical literature of what could reasonably be termed "psychogenic dyspareunia." Psychological and relational factors are important mediators of the experience of dyspareunia, but there are precious few data indicating that they give rise to the disorder.

Vaginismus is described as a recurrent or persistent involuntary spasm of the musculature of the outer third of the vagina that interferes with sexual intercourse. Interestingly, no mental health professional is in a position to verify this uniquely physical criterion appearing in a mental health manual. Furthermore, no woman presents clinically with this description. Typically the woman with vaginismus presents with intense fear of vaginal penetration, descriptions of penetration attempts as painful and distressing, and assertions that penetration is either impossible or close to impossible much of the time. Many of these women have similar fears and avoidance of gynecological exams. In fact, the vaginal muscle spasm definition of vaginismus appears to be based primarily on expert opinion, as there is no empirical evidence to support vaginal/pelvic muscle spasm as the defining characteristic of vaginismus (Binik, 2010b).

Recent research has cast doubt on our ability to reliably distinguish vaginismus from certain types of dyspareunia (e.g., PVD). They both share reports of pain with sexual intercourse and with gynecological examinations, and both are characterized by an avoidance of penetration. It could be that vaginismus exists on the extreme end of a behavioral/affective continuum of dyspareunia. The one distinguishing characteristic may be fear and distress about vaginal penetration and pain, with women who typically receive the diagnosis of vaginismus suffering more from both (Reissing, Binik, Khalife, Cohen, & Amsel, 2004).

Genito-pelvic pain/penetration disorder is the new diagnostic category proposed for the DSM-5 (American Psychiatric Association, 2012). Originally, the radical recommendation was that this diagnostic category be entirely removed from the sexual disorders section of the DSM and be reclassified into the pain disorders section of the manual. The rationale was that the data support a conceptualization of dyspareunia and vaginismus as pain disorders that happen to interfere with sex, much as other pain disorders interfere with sex and other aspects of daily living. Calling them sexual pain disorders and classifying them with the other sexual dysfunctions inaccurately elevates the role of sex in their development. Furthermore, the new category would subsume the current diagnoses of dyspareunia and vaginismus, with the rationale that there is no current empirical basis for the differentiation between these two diagnoses. The latest draft of the proposal (last updated July 29, 2011) appears to indicate that genito-pelvic pain/penetration disorder, if adopted, will continue to be classified as a sexual dysfunction. The proposed criteria require persistent or recurrent difficulties with at least one of the following: inability to have vaginal intercourse/penetration, vulvovaginal or pelvic pain during penetration attempts, fear or anxiety about pain or penetration, tensing of pelvic floor muscles during vaginal penetration attempts. As in the case of the other two proposed categories, the distress criterion and onset sub-type are retained, while a list of specifiers is added to cover contextual influences.

1.3   Epidemiology

After decades of reliance on convenience and clinical samples, large-scale national and cross-national epidemiological surveys providing valuable prevalence data have been conducted in the last 15 years. Other than variations in the wording of question items, there are two important points to consider when interpreting the data across studies. The first of these is the time frame covered by the question. Some questions inquire whether the symptom lasted at least 1 month, while others cover at least 6 months, or a period of several months in the last year. Answers vary significantly according to the time frame indicated. The DSM-IV-TR's use of "persistent and recurrent" in Criterion A for all sexual dysfunctions leaves undefined how long the problem has to have existed for a diagnosis to be made (the proposed revisions to the DSM are more specific about duration and frequency of symptoms).

The second important point to consider is whether the women surveyed are distressed by the problem or whether the problem is causing relationship discord (Criterion B of all sexual dysfunctions in the DSM-IV). As we shall see, reports of sexual problems with associated distress are far less prevalent than reports of sexual symptoms without concomitant distress. Although the absence of distress should preclude a diagnosis as per the DSM-IV, it remains informative to consider women's reports of their sexuality, whether or not distress is present.

1.3.1   Low Desire or Interest in Sex

Across studies, low sexual desire has been shown to be highly prevalent in women. Because of the potential of gender desire discrepancies contributing to the inflation of HSDD diagnoses in women, data for men are here reported when possible. In the National Health and Social Life Survey (NHSLS), 27% to 32% of sexually active women ($n = 1,749$) and 13% to 17% of men ($n = 1,410$) in the United States aged 18 to 59 reported lack of interest in sex over several months or more in the prior year (Laumann, Paik, & Rosen, 1999). In the National Survey of Sexual Attitudes and Lifestyles (Natsal), 40.6% of 5,530 women in Britain aged 16 to 44 reported lack of interest in sex of 1 month's duration over the prior year, in contrast to 17.1% of men surveyed (Mercer et al., 2003). Lack of interest in sex lasting at least 6 months in the past year was reported by 10.2% of women and 1.8% of men. Although the numbers dropped considerably when the time frame was extended, low sexual desire remained the most common complaint in women in the Natsal, as well as in the Global Study of Sexual Attitudes and Behaviors (GSSAB). The latter found a prevalence of 26% to 43% for lack of interest in sex among those sexually active in their sample of 13,882 women from 29 countries, aged 40 to 80 years (Laumann et al., 2005), compared with a prevalence of 13% to 28% in men.

Clearly, many women report low levels of sexual desire, but we do not generally know how women arrive at their sexual desire self-assessment. No study has systematically investigated what or who women are comparing with when they rate their desire levels. Are they comparing their level of desire to an earlier, more intense, level, or are they comparing their desire with that of men and consequently judging their desire levels accordingly, even when they do not care about the difference? Nicolson and Burr (2003) have suggested that the sexology literature has promoted the existence of a mythical standard of female sexuality against which women measure themselves. Without this assumption regarding how much desire is normative or "healthy," perhaps fewer women would report low desire. In any case, it is essential to review associated distress if we are to estimate the prevalence of HSDD in women.

Table 3 presents prevalence rates for low desire compared with those for low desire associated with distress, in studies that investigated both. Basically, the inclusion of distress yields ranges that are half the size of those for reports of low desire that do not take distress into account (with distress: 8–26% versus without distress: 16–55%). Nonetheless, the number of women across

Prevalence of self-reported low desire is very high, but half of these women are not distressed by their desire levels

Table 3
Comparison of Prevalence Rates of Low Desire to Prevalence Rates of Low Desire With Associated Distress in Women

Study	Female sample size and characteristics	Country	Age	Low desire (%)	Low desire + distress (%)[a]
Fugl-Meyer & Fugl-Meyer (1999)	N = 1,335	Sweden	18–74	34	15
Oberg et al. (2004)	N = 1,056 who had intercourse at least once in past year	Sweden	19–65	29[b]	15[c]
Leiblum et al. (2006)	N = 952 surgically/ naturally postmenopausal, sexually active	USA	20–70	24–36	9–26
Dennerstein et al. (2006)	N = 2,467 women, sexually active	France, Italy Germany, UK	20–70	16–46	7–16
West et al. (2008)	N = 755 premenopausal, 552 naturally menopausal, 637 surgically menopausal, in relationship for at least 3 months	USA	30–70	36	8
Witting et al. (2009)	N = 5,463, partnered sexual activity over past 4 weeks	Finland	18–49	55	23
Shifren et al. (2008)	N = 13,581	USA	18–102	34	10

Note. [a]Desire and distress were variably assessed across studies. [b]This prevalence rate is for what the authors described as manifest low desire (low desire quite often, nearly all, or all of the time). [c]This prevalence rate is for low desire and what the authors described as manifest distress (concomitant personal distress quite often, nearly all, or all of the time).

studies reporting low desire and the associated distress necessary for a DSM-IV diagnosis remains fairly high. In their review of 11 studies inquiring about desire, arousal, orgasm, and pain, Hayes, Bennett, Fairley, and Dennerstein (2006) found that 64% of all women with any sexual difficulty specified low sexual desire to be the presumed cause. HSDD is thus likely the most prevalent of the female sexual dysfunctions by any definition and the most highly associated with other impairments in sexual function.

The prevalence of SAD is unknown. None of the aforementioned population-based epidemiological studies asked about sexual aversion specifically. One study of 382 undergraduates conducted over 20 years ago reported a prevalence of approximately 10% using a specific measure of sexual aversion that assessed fear of AIDS, social evaluation, pregnancy, and sexual trauma (Katz, Gipson, Kearl, & Kriskovich, 1989). Considering the severity of the requisite symptoms for a diagnosis of SAD, that estimate now seems high and may have been strongly related to the HIV epidemic at the time the study was conducted. It is also hard to know how many cases of SAD are diagnosed as HSDD. The scarce literature available does, however, support a higher prevalence of this disorder in women than in men (Brotto, 2010).

1.3.2   Arousal Difficulties

There are a number of problems in assessing population estimates of FSAD. In terms of DSM-IV-TR criteria, one would have to rule out cases in which the FSAD could reasonably be attributed to another sexual dysfunction and/or the physiological effects of a substance/medication or a general medical condition. In terms of other sexual dysfunctions, it is easy to imagine that HSDD might easily result in FSAD, and women are likely to report lack of desire as the more prominent complaint. After all, most women with low desire would consider lack of arousal to be a secondary problem. Although menopause-related changes arguably do not constitute a medical condition, they have certainly been documented to have an impact on genital tissue thickness and elasticity, as well as on lubrication. In addition, FSAD would not be a reasonable diagnosis in a woman who does not receive adequate sexual stimulation. Yet prevalence studies rarely inquire about the competence of sexual stimulation. Most studies simply inquire about lubrication (not swelling). To complicate matters, different studies inquire about lubrication problems in reference to different time frames.

In all of these large-scale studies combined, the range of women reporting lubrication problems during any time frame (from the previous month to several months in the past year) is 2.6% to 31.2% (Graham, 2010a). The range is large and appears to depend on time frame and age of respondents. Although lubrication problems appear to increase with age, only a handful of epidemiological studies have recruited postmenopausal women. The GSSAB by Laumann et al. (2005) specifically targeted sexually active (intercourse at least once in the previous year) women aged 40–80 years from 29 countries. They found 16.1% to 37.9% of women reporting lubrication difficulties. Age was related to lubrication difficulties in almost all countries. Thus, lubrication difficulties appear to be relatively common, but they may be intricately entwined with other sexual dysfunctions, age, and the adequacy of sexual stimulation.

1.3.3   Difficulties With Orgasm

A review of 11 surveys using nationally representative samples found a wide range for women reporting difficulties with orgasm (Graham, 2010b). As in the case of desire and arousal, studies have varied in terms of how questions were asked, the time frame involved, and the extent to which distress about the problems was taken into account. The number of women across these studies endorsing complete inability to achieve orgasm (with or/and without a partner) has ranged from approximately 10% to 34%. The number of women endorsing difficulties (although not impossibility of) reaching orgasm have ranged from 11% to 30%. In a cross-national older sample of women aged 40–80 years, inability to reach orgasm ranged from approximately 18% to 41% (Laumann et al., 2005).

Results to date indicate that approximately half (or less) of women who report difficulty attaining orgasm appear to be distressed about it. Yet again, absence of distress appears to be the only criterion that stands between many women and a DSM-IV diagnosis. On the other hand, this is of little clinical relevance as women who are not distressed about their sexual function are unlikely to seek treatment.

1.3.4   Pain With Intercourse

Determining the true prevalence of dyspareunia and vaginismus is plagued by the same methodological difficulties as those afflicting the epidemiology of the other sexual dysfunctions in women. The data differ depending on the time frame you inquire about, the frequency and intensity of the pain, and whether or not you are going to exclude medical conditions of unknown etiology with few, if any, physiological manifestations (e.g., PVD). The difficulty distinguishing dyspareunia from vaginismus also muddies the picture. When Laumann, Gagnon, Michael and Michaels (1994) asked women aged 18–59 if they had experienced physical pain during intercourse over a period of several months in the past year, 14.4% said yes. Surprisingly, the age group in that study with the highest prevalence was women aged 18–24, 21.5% of whom endorsed experiencing this problem. It is suspected that the most common cause of premenopausal dyspareunia (and possibly of vaginismus) is PVD (Harlow, Wise, & Stewart, 2001).

The prevalence of dyspareunia is highest in young women, and its most common cause is PVD

One could argue that women with PVD should not receive a DSM-IV diagnosis of dyspareunia because it constitutes a general medical condition. However, this type of exclusionary criterion remains stuck in dualistic notions about our ability to differentiate between psychological and physical factors. PVD is diagnosed by a particular pain profile (tenderness at 4, 6, and 8 o'clock on the vulvar vestibule) and rarely manifests other physical indicators, with the exception of pelvic floor muscle hypertonicity. On the other hand, PVD has been associated with a significant number of psychological correlates (pain hypervigilance and catastrophization) that are important to treatment.

Pain with intercourse is a fairly prevalent female sexual complaint and perhaps the one in which distress is the most commonly experienced. Limiting the diagnosis of either dyspareunia or vaginismus to women in whom the pain appears to be exclusively psychogenic is likely to be pointless, primarily because of our inability to make that determination, and because most cases of sexual pain appear to have a physical etiology that is highly influenced by psychological factors.

1.4   Course and Prognosis

The course and prognosis of sexual dysfunctions in women, whether or not they receive treatment, is believed to be highly variable. This is especially true of acquired rather than lifelong sexual dysfunctions.

Untreated course of some female sexual dysfunctions can be variable but others, such as dyspareunia, are mostly chronic

In terms of HSDD, the lifelong form of the dysfunction usually has a perceived onset at some point in adolescence, when sexual feelings arise or fail to arise. Women with lifelong HSDD report never having felt a motivation to seek sex or never having been interested in responding to sexual advances, other than for instrumental (nonsexual) reasons. The more frequent presentation is the acquired form of HSDD which manifests after a period of self-reported adequate desire. Acquired HSDD consequently appears in adulthood. Although loss or decreases in desire have been associated with a number of physical, psychological, or relational factors, a significant number of women report having no idea why their sexual desire faded (Sims & Meana, 2010).

Prognosis in the absence of treatment is impossible to ascertain, because of its variable nature. Reasonable assumptions are that lifelong HSDD is unlikely to change without intervention and that acquired HSDD is likely to resolve if the conditions that gave rise to it resolve. These latter conditions, such as entrenched relationship dynamics, may be, however, quite immutable without intervention. Equally likely is the return of HSDD if other conditions develop that are likely to impact negatively on sexual desire (e.g., symptoms of depression or anxiety, self-esteem deficits, body image concerns). Because of the high comorbidity between FSAD and HSDD, their course and prognosis are generally assumed to be similar, barring age and menopause-related changes that may have a direct impact on genital tissue and lubrication in the case of FSAD.

There is insufficient research on SAD to assert a course and/or prognosis. Theories of SAD as a conditioned aversion, however, indicate an acquired course such that sexual stimuli were at some point paired with the experience of pain or trauma. If SAD in fact follows the course of most phobias, then one would expect the course to be relatively chronic, if not increasingly severe, over time. Likewise, prognosis is likely to be relatively dire without direct intervention. Even with intervention, the prognosis is not as good as we would hope. As in the case of most phobias, interventions have been shown to effectively reduce fear and anxiety, but they do not generally engender an affection or passion for the once-feared stimulus. In the case of fear of flying, being able to tolerate flying without panic symptoms or catastrophizing cognitions would be considered a treatment success. The patient does not have to love flying or become a pilot, for the intervention to be deemed effective. Just getting on the plane and making it through the flight without a panic attack would be considered good enough.

Clearly the bar has to be set a little higher in the case of sexual aversion. The ultimate aim of sex (other than procreation) is pleasure and the feeling of closeness and connectedness with a partner. It is important for clinicians to appreciate that simply tolerating the activity is unlikely to be considered a treatment success either by a client or by her partner.

Ascertaining the course of FOD is complicated by the fact that a woman's first orgasm can occur anytime from late childhood to advanced adulthood. Unlike in men, whose first orgasm most often occurs around puberty, women may be perfectly capable of achieving orgasm yet only have their first orgasm as adults, either because they did not masturbate or because they had partnered sex that was unskilled. As aforementioned, it is not unusual in clinical settings to encounter women who believe (or whose partners believe) they are anorgasmic because they do not reach orgasm through intercourse. In these cases the supposed FOD is simply a function of failing to receive adequate clitoral stimulation, either during penetration or through manual or oral stimulation. In cases such as these, what looks like lifelong FOD can easily be resolved with competent stimulation.

The prognosis for both lifelong and acquired FOD, without direct intervention, thus depends on the cause of the FOD and the likelihood that causative factors will resolve. For example, if a skillful sexual partner replaces an unskillful sexual partner or if a woman takes it upon herself to learn what type of stimulation works for her, the prognosis may be good. On the other hand, if the FOD is acquired and appears concomitant with vulvovaginal atrophy, the prognosis may be worse with or without intervention.

Left untreated, the course of the sexual pain disorders appears to be mostly chronic. This is probably attributable to two factors. In the case of dyspareunia, there is little evidence of spontaneous remission of the hyperinnervation of vulvar tissue associated with the most common type of premenopausal dyspareunia, PVD. In the case of postmenopausal dyspareunia attributable to vaginal atrophy, there is similarly little reason to believe that the situation would improve on its own. Actually, the theoretically supported expectation is that, without intervention, the sexual pain disorders are likely to worsen with time. First, there is the possible tissue damage and irritation effected by penetration in the absence of lubrication and in the presence of hypertonicity. Then there is the classical conditioning of sex as a pain stimulus. Over time, the repeated pairing of pain (not to mention anxiety and relationship discord) with sex (in both dyspareunia and vaginismus) can turn sexual stimuli into conditioned pain (physical and emotional) stimuli. The prognosis with treatment is better, but the efficacy of treatments for the sexual pain disorders is variable. Some women experience great relief or total resolution of the problem, while for others, the best-case scenario is effective pain management, rather than pain resolution.

1.5   Differential Diagnosis

The main differential diagnoses in the sexual dysfunctions for women are sexual dysfunction due to a general medical condition, substance-induced sexual dysfunction, or other Axis I disorder.

Sexual dysfunction due to a general medical disorder is a problematic differential diagnosis because it rests on a dichotomous notion of sexual dysfunction being easily attributable to either physical factors or psychological ones. The reality is that many clients are likely to have both physical and psychological involvement. Even when a general medical condition is the obvious source of the difficulty, there are likely to be a number of psychological sequelae (e.g., anxiety, shame, self-esteem concerns, relationship difficulties) that have developed over time and have a very real impact on dysfunction symptoms. Resolving the originating physical problem does not always result in the resolution of the sexual symptoms. In other words, the factors that gave rise to the problem may be different from the ones that maintain it. Thus, one has to assess whether a general medical condition is involved in the dysfunction and ensure that it is being addressed. However, the discovery of a medical condition is not as much a differential diagnosis as it is important information to be integrated into the treatment plan.

In the case of HSDD, neurological, hormonal, and metabolic abnormalities may impair desire. Sexual aversion has not generally been associated with general medical conditions. FSAD, on the other hand, has been associated with menopausal or postmenopausal reduction in estrogen levels, as well as any number of medical problems that can impact genital tissue. FSAD and FOD can also manifest as a side effect of treatments for any number of diseases, including cancers. Although the most common medical condition associated with the sexual pain disorders is PVD, the sexual pain disorders have also been linked to a wide range of medical conditions and postmenopausal changes in genital tissue. See Section 3.1.1 and Table 4 for general medical conditions associated with female sexual dysfunction. It is important to keep in mind that the impact of general medical conditions on sexual function is often more than physical. Being diagnosed with a serious disease or having body-altering surgeries can have psychological effects (e.g., anxiety, depression, body image disturbances) whose impact on sexual function can far outweigh physical limitations.

Theoretically, ruling out substance-induced sexual dysfunction should be less complicated if the patient is in a position to actively test whether the dysfunction occurs exclusively when the substance is being used. The problem is that the substances that feature most prominently in sexuality-related clinical practice are prescription medications that constitute important treatment for some other physical or mental health condition (e.g., selective serotonin reuptake inhibitors and antihypertensive medications). When discontinuation is not an option, one can only experiment with different products and dosages to try to find the optimal balance. Sometimes this is possible, sometimes it is not. Sometimes it works, and sometimes it does not. In these cases it is also difficult to determine whether the sexual symptoms are truly attributable to the medication, to the underlying disease, or to neither. (See Section 3.1.1 and Table 4 for classes of substances and medications associated with female sexual dysfunction.)

Determining whether the sexual dysfunction is better accounted for by another Axis I disorder (other than other sexual dysfunctions) can be challenging. Except in instances wherein the sexual dysfunction clearly fluctuates with an Axis I disorder, it is nearly impossible to determine if the sexual symptoms are primarily a consequence of the latter. Because many Axis I disorders can have a significant impact on the accuracy of cognitions, relying on a client's assessment of the onset of sexual symptoms can also be misleading. In the case of SAD, the symptomatology may meet criteria for specific phobia, but as the DSM-IV currently stands, the SAD diagnosis is made in its stead.

Dyspareunia is the only sexual dysfunction in the DSM-IV that has another sexual dysfunction as an exclusionary criterion. If the pain with intercourse is believed to be a consequence of vaginismus, then vaginismus is the diagnosis. Given our current difficulty in distinguishing between these two sexual dysfunctions, determining whether a patient has dyspareunia or vaginismus is also challenging. The combination of extreme fear, anxiety, and avoidance of penetration and gynecological exams is probably the most reliable discriminating factor between these two current diagnostic categories. Even if dyspareunia and vaginismus end up being merged in the DSM-5, these characteristics are likely to distinguish between two types of women experiencing pain with intercourse.

In summary, the types of exclusions that the DSM-IV states as the bases of differential diagnoses are, from a clinical practice standpoint, best regarded as important specifiers to consider and integrate into treatment plans. Assessing for general medical conditions, substances and medications, and the presence of other Axis I disorders is of paramount importance to the multidisciplinary treatment of sexual dysfunctions in women. However, it is only rarely that the existence of any one of these factors will render sex-focused interventions superfluous. Sexual problems generally have complicated multifactorial etiologies that require the clinician to target all of them simultaneously, instead of trying to determine the rank order of their causal force.

1.6   Comorbidities

Although there are multiple risk factors for sexual dysfunctions (see Section 3), the comorbidity of most relevance to the treatment of any sexual dysfunction is the existence of another sexual dysfunction either in the client or in her partner. At least in clinical settings, sexual problems in women tend to affect all phases of the sexual response. Starting at one end of the linear sexual response model, it is not difficult to imagine how low or no desire might lead to arousal difficulties which might lead to difficulty achieving orgasm. At the other end, if a woman starts to develop difficulties with orgasm, one might imagine that desire for sexual activity might also wane (although it is important to note that sexual satisfaction in women is not as closely tied to orgasm as it is in men). If the sexual experience culminates in pain, as in the case of dyspareunia and vaginismus, problems with desire and arousal are likely.

In women with more than one sexual dysfunction, determining which came first is difficult and may not be important to treatment

Many studies have found evidence for the high comorbidity of sexual problems and dysfunctions in women. Clinical samples of women with a primary diagnosis of HSDD have shown that up to 41% reported at least one other sexual dysfunction, while 18% had 3 concurrent sexual dysfunction diagnoses (Segraves & Segraves, 1991). Surveys of large community samples in North America and Europe also show high comorbidity rates for all of the sexual dysfunctions, regardless of age or hormonal status. Desire, arousal, and orgasm problems appear to have the strongest associations (for a review, see van Lankveld, 2008). The sexual pain disorders have lower associations with the other dysfunctions (although generally still significant), perhaps because pain is perceived as an interloper symptom that is not directly related to the sexual response. This supports the idea that dyspareunia and vaginismus may be more akin to pain disorders than to sexual dysfunctions.

Given the high comorbidity of the sexual dysfunctions, it can be difficult to establish which condition is the primary problem (except possibly in the case of the sexual pain disorders). As in the case of the differential diagnoses, the point may be moot considering that typically all aspects of sexual function need to be addressed simultaneously in order for treatment to be effective. Even if intercourse pain is the primary culprit, the situation can only be helped by attempts to increase desire, arousal, and orgasmic capacity. The one exception to this might be SAD, which can sometimes hide quite surreptitiously under an initial presentation of HSDD. Some women are embarrassed to admit their feelings of revulsion, or fear that their open expression would hurt their partner.

Thus, women with SAD can present with low or no sexual desire. Typically, however, their avoidance of sexual activity is more pronounced that that of women with HSDD, and the aversion surfaces quite dramatically when treatment components that require sexual contact are introduced. Distinguishing between HSDD and SAD is important, as the treatment for SAD will have to focus on fear and anxiety, neither of which is as pronounced in HSDD.

In any case, the high comorbidity rates for the sexual dysfunctions in women should alert the clinician to engage in a full assessment of all aspects of sexual function. The ultimate aim is to devise a treatment plan that simultaneously targets all components of the woman's sexual response. Data clearly indicate that the female sexual response is not easily divisible.

2

Theories and Models of Sexual Dysfunction

Much of sex research has lacked a strong theoretical basis. From Kinsey's interviews, to Masters and Johnson's physiological measurements, to today's deliberations about what constitutes a sexual dysfunction diagnosis, our data collection efforts have outshone our attempts at organizing these data into a unifying theory of how sex functions and how it "dysfunctions." This theoretical void has only recently started to be more vigorously targeted. There are now a number of general theoretical models that attempt to account for a broad range of sexual variations. The empirical testing of these models is in its nascence, although growing.

Different theories have their unique emphases. There are, however, three consistent themes running through all current attempts to provide unifying accounts of how sexual problems might arise and be maintained in both men and women: *diversity* (individual/gender differences), the *integration of mind and body*, and the *multidetermined nature* of sexual function (biological, psychological, social, economic, and cultural contributors). *Complexity* is thus the operative word. None of the theories make single causal pathway claims about sexual dysfunction, and little attempt is made to distinguish etiological factors from mediating ones. This probably reflects more the state of the science than a deliberate strategy. Below is a brief and selective review of recent theories that address how sexual function can go awry as a function of multiple components within the complex schema that encompasses sexuality.

All current models acknowledge the diversity of sexual experience, the mind-body integration, and the multidetermined nature of sexual function

2.1   Barlow's Cognitive-Affective Model

A negative feedback loop was the central concept in Barlow's original cognitive-affective model of how sexual dysfunctions develop (Barlow, 1986). Sexual situations automatically represent demands on sexual performance. In the sexually dysfunctional individual, this demand triggers a process of anxious apprehension whereby attention shifts away from erotic cues to negative, internal self-evaluative ones that in turn interfere with performance and result in even greater apprehension and anxiety. Untreated, that negative feedback loop has a tendency to be reinforced over time, and sexual dysfunction can become entrenched.

Barlow's original model was developed from research on men, and it did not account for biological predispositions to dysfunction. It has since been modified to integrate new data. However, the original centrality of the impact of distraction from erotic cues and attention on anxiety-provoking cues remains. The model has considerable empirical support, although research on women has made us reevaluate what sexual performance means to them and how central a concern that is or is not for women.

2.2   Dual-Control Model

The dual-control model posits that the sexual response in any given individual and any given situation is contingent on the balance of two systems with neurobiological substrates: the sexual excitation system and the sexual inhibition system (Bancroft & Janssen, 2000). Both are adaptive in that excitation propels to sexual activity (procreation) while inhibition reduces the likelihood of the sexual response when it may not be in the individual's best short-term or long-term interests (risk reduction). While acknowledging the influence of relational, social, and contextual factors on the sexual response, this model proposes that the effects of sexual stimulation will ultimately depend on an individual's neurobiological characteristics. Preliminary data suggest that there are individual and gender differences in the propensity for excitation and inhibition. Questionnaire data suggest that women manifest more inhibition and less excitation than men (Milhausen, Graham, Sanders, Yarber, & Maitland, 2010).

In this model, sexual problems might arise when there is an imbalance in either the excitation or the inhibition systems or in their relationship to each other. Individuals with a low propensity for excitation and/or a high propensity for inhibition would be more susceptible to experiencing sexual difficulties (the inverse might result in hypersexuality and/or high risk sexual behaviors). However, the indication of gender differences in propensities for excitation and inhibition alerts us to the fact that determinations of whether an imbalance exists would have to be made relative to gender. Otherwise, women would de facto be expected to experience more sexual problems than men. Certainly, the epidemiological data assert that women report lower sexual desire, arousal, and orgasm frequency than do men. The question is determining when those lower levels are a problem (other than a discrepancy one). This concern underlies the insistence of some to maintain the distress criterion in diagnostic classifications.

2.3   Sexual Tipping Point® Model

The Sexual Tipping Point® model of Perelman (2009) also uses the concept of balance to delineate the development of sexual dysfunction. It posits that at any given point for any one individual, there will be a threshold for the expression or triggering of any phase of the sexual response, from desire to arousal to orgasm. Excitatory physiological, psychosocial, relational, and cultural factors weigh in against parallel inhibitory ones. Depending on the relative weight of the positive and negative factors, the balance will tip in favor of a sexual response, a neutral response, or a sexually inhibiting response. This process is conceived as a dynamic one in which the combination of factors that will tip the scale in favor of a positive or negative response will vary across situations and across the life span. Because the tipping point is determined by the weight of multiple factors encompassing both the physical as well as the sociopsychological, this model actively argues for the multidisciplinary treatment of sexual dysfunction. Perelman suggests that multidisciplinary treatment might be even more important for sexual dysfunction in women, as psychological and relational factors may carry more weight and thus have more potential to enhance and disrupt sexual function. No research study to date has directly tested this model, although existing data support its general premise.

2.4   Intersystems Approach

The intersystems approach to conceptualizing the possible causes and mediators of sexual dysfunction focuses on the interactivity of three systems – individual, interactional, and intergenerational (Weeks & Cross, 2004). Although this approach grew out of theories of marital and family therapy, it nonetheless incorporates physiological factors as possible sources of sexual problems. In an attempt to balance both individual and relational concerns, the framework proposes five dimensions of relevance to the conceptualization and treatment of sexual dysfunction: biological/medical, psychological, dyadic relationship, family of origin, and sociocultural/religious/historical. This approach consequently promotes the multidisciplinary treatment of sexual dysfunction and argues for comprehensive theoretical frameworks that encompass the richness of, and thus varied, potential complications in the sexual lives of clients. Here too, data supporting this model have not been particularly forthcoming as research design is particularly challenging with such holistic frameworks.

2.5   New View Approach

Concerns about reductionism in the study and treatment of sexuality, the increasing medicalization of sexual variation, and a perceived failure of sexology to account for the sociopolitical pressures on women's sexuality led Leonore Tiefer and colleagues to propose a new nonsymptom-focused classification scheme for women's sexual dysfunction (Working Group on a New View of Women's Sexual Problems, 2000). The New View was organized around the potential causes of women's sexual problems. It proposes that individuals should identify their own sexual problems through the assertion of "discontent or dissatisfaction with any emotional, physical, or relational aspect of the sexual experience." Rather than defining sexual dysfunction through a list of predetermined symptoms that provide a normative definition of what should be experienced, this model lets the client decide what is and is not normal for him or her, what is and is not a problem.

Within this depathologizing framework, sexual problems can be attributed to (1) sociocultural, political, or economic factors, (2) partner or relationship,

(3) psychological factors, and/or (4) medical factors. The New View approach shares with other models the view that sexual problems are multidetermined. However, it is unique in its resistance to the imposition of definitions of sexual dysfunction on individuals. Leaving it up to the woman to determine if she has a problem, the New View then turns in a more pointed fashion than other models to the potential causal force of women's sociopolitical and cultural disadvantages. To date, there has only been one direct empirical test of this classification system whereby women's open-ended responses about their sexual complaints were examined for their fit to the New View categories (Nicholls, 2008). Although results supported the model, more research is needed, as is the case with all of the other models.

2.6   Summary and Integration of Models

Looking over existing theories and models of how sexual difficulties can arise, one can easily get the sense that these theories have thrown in "everything but the kitchen sink." Although that might be a fair assessment, its negative connotation is not. That an individual's sexual response is affected by multiple factors is no surprise. Although the scientific method is generally driven to isolate specific causal factors, sexuality is rarely amenable to that narrow a strategy. Clinical practice almost never is. It is likely that, in any given case of sexual difficulty, some factors will be more important than others. Yet, determining the relative importance of the multitude of influences on a sexual response can be very difficult and, most often, simply impossible. As clinicians engaged in dutiful comprehensive assessment, we may get a sense of the relative contribution of factors to our clients' sexual problems, but ultimately, our treatment will likely to have to address multiple factors equally vigorously.

Our clients' bodies, thoughts, emotions, behavior, and relationship dynamics and skills are all important targets for treatment. The following section will focus on empirically and theoretically supported risk factors for specific sexual dysfunctions. In doing so, the field of causes and mediators will narrow somewhat. The bad news is that it remains complicated. The good news is that all clinical psychologists, not just sex therapists, have training relevant to many aspects of their clients' lives likely to be involved in either the development or the maintenance of sexual disturbances. They also have training in the cognitive and behavioral interventions that are most empirically supported in the treatment of sexual problems.

3

Diagnosis and Treatment Indications

3.1 Risk and Dysfunction-Maintaining Factors

Given the significant overlap in potential etiologies for female sexual dysfunctions, as well as their high comorbidity, risk factors across dysfunctions should be considered simultaneously. In terms of assessment, this strategy can alert the clinician to the possible existence of complications (and/or dysfunctions) over and above the one the client presents with. In concert with the biopsychosocial model to which most extant theories of sexual function and dysfunction adhere, there are three major categories of risk factors that are important to consider in treatment planning: biomedical, psychological, and relational/social. The coverage of each of these categories in this text is by no means exhaustive. It is based on the most common presentations and those for which we have the most empirical support. However, it is important to keep in mind that sexual function remains an underinvestigated aspect of medical conditions, psychological well-being, and relational/social adjustment. Clinicians are urged to be expansive in their consideration of risk factors and feel free to move beyond the necessarily selective list that follows.

3.1.1 Biomedical

Age
On one level, age is a biological factor. Our bodies change with time and in ways that can affect sexual function. On another, age is a complex psychosocial factor that encompasses a number of life-span phases characterized by varyingly focused cognitions, emotions, and relationships that can also affect sexual function. As it is the easiest data point to collect, we have a fair amount of information on the association of age with sexual problems. The interpretation of that association is another, more complicated, story.

Cross-national epidemiological studies indicate that, for the most part, sexual function declines with age in both women and men (Hayes & Dennerstein, 2005; Lewis et al., 2010,). Cross-study inconsistencies in collecting data on the distress criterion, however, make it less clear whether the prevalence of DSM-IV–defined sexual dysfunctions increase as women get older. Rates of low desire appear to double in women aged 50–65 compared with women under 50. These rates double again in the 66–74-year-old age group, although there appears to be some indication that distress associated with low desire declines with age. Lubrication insufficiency, such as would qualify for Criterion A in the diagnosis of FSAD, is also more common in older women. The data on orgasmic dysfunction is not as consistent, although it also points to an increase in orgasm difficulties (delay and intensity) with age. The one exception to the age/sexual dysfunction concordance may be the sexual pain disorders: dyspareunia and vaginismus. Although vulvovaginal atrophy associated with menopause can make penetration uncomfortable, severe pain with intercourse appears to be more prevalent in younger women.

Ageist and sexist social norms can have a negative impact on the sexual function of older women

Age might, however, be a risk factor for decreases in sexual function in women independent of menopause-associated changes. Older women face a number of relational and social challenges which can have a negative impact on sexual function over and above age-related changes in endocrine function or general health. Their general societal devaluation as sexual beings is one of these. On the other hand, the importance of sex to women appears to decrease with age, thus leaving open the possibility that decreases in function are not necessarily experienced as problematic.

Hormones

Both estrogens and androgens appear to play important roles in the sexual function of women, although it is not always easy to establish in exactly what ways. One reason for the difficulty lies in the fact that both of these classes of hormones can have a positive impact on mood, which can in turn positively affect sexual function. Another difficulty lies in the fact that it can be difficult to tease apart the effects of estrogen and androgen in women, as the former is synthesized from the latter. Hormonal deficits have been linked, although inconsistently, to reductions in desire, lubrication, orgasmic capacity and intensity, and to dyspareunia.

In terms of estrogens, the data have been gathered mostly from the study of menopause and associated treatments. This research indicates that estrogens have a generally positive impact on women's sexual function given that the administration of exogenous estrogen after menopause tends to produce generally positive effects. The clearest impact of estrogen replacement therapy, however, is on genital tissue and lubrication. Thus, research indicates that estrogen deficiency is a bigger risk factor for lubrication problems and for pain with intercourse than it is for low sexual desire. In premenopausal women, there is unlikely to be an estrogen-related explanation for sexual problems.

Testosterone appears to have a stronger impact on the general sexual function of women than does estrogen

Although women have, on average, circulating levels of testosterone one tenth those of men, at certain critical levels, androgens may play a more direct a role in sexual dysfunction than do estrogens. There is, however, great variability in women's sensitivity and responsivity to testosterone, making it impossible to determine a normative, critical level under which sexual dysfunction would be expected. Variations in androgen levels in healthy premenopausal women do not have a strong and consistent association with sexual desire or arousal. In some studies, androgen levels have not been found to predict sexual desire in women at all (Davis, Davison, Donath, & Bell, 2005). In addition, sexual desire is not strongly associated with elevated testosterone around ovulation, and supraphysiological androgen levels pharmacologically induced in healthy women have not been shown to have a significant impact on sexual desire. On the other hand, there are reports of women on steroidal contraceptives, known to reduce free testosterone, who complain of reductions in sexual desire.

The story is simpler when we turn away from normal hormonal variations to clear cases of androgen insufficiency. Low androgen levels in women are most commonly associated with natural or surgical menopause (bilateral oophorectomy) or other medical procedures (e.g., chemotherapy or radiotherapy) and conditions (e.g., adrenal disease) that can reduce or eliminate androgen production. Low sexual desire and orgasm difficulties are common sequelae of these processes. Further proof of the role of androgens comes from an increasingly convincing body of data showing significant improvements in sexual function with androgen replacement therapy (Apperloo, Van der Stege, Hoek, & Weijmar Schultz, 2003). Exogenous testosterone largely restores the sexual desire, arousal, and orgasmic capacity of these women.

Although less often considered in relation to sexual function, prolactin, a peptide hormone produced in the pituitary gland and known to regulate lactation, has also been associated with sexual interest in clinical populations. High serum levels of prolactin (hyperprolactinemia) have been associated with low sexual interest in chronic hemodialysis patients and in individuals with pituitary tumors, as well as in pregnant women and women who are lactating. However, much as with androgens, sexual desire does not seem to vary as a function of prolactin in healthy populations. Women reporting low desire who are neither ill nor pregnant or lactating do not differ from women with no such sexual complaints, in terms of their prolactin levels.

In summary, hormone deficiencies or (overproduction) are risk factors for sexual dysfunctions, but there are important caveats to keep in mind. In the healthy premenopausal woman (who is neither pregnant nor lactating), hormone levels are an unlikely single cause for sexual dysfunction. Furthermore, the administration of testosterone to healthy premenopausal women has currently unknown but potentially serious health risks. On the other hand, if the premenopausal woman complaining of low desire is on oral contraceptives, it may be worth considering their potential role in her decreased libido and arousal. In terms of the naturally or surgically menopausal woman, hormone deficiencies are a likely risk factor for sexual difficulties ranging from low desire to dyspareunia.

Hormones are unlikely to underlie sexual problems in healthy, premenopausal women, but there are individual sensitivities to oral contraceptives

Genes

The study of genetic influences on the development of sexual dysfunction is in its infancy, but there are some intriguing results worth considering. A Finnish study of over 6,000 female twins found modest evidence for a genetic susceptibility to sexual dysfunction, although individual factors appeared to be much stronger predictors of the development of dysfunction (Witting et al., 2009). Other research is indicating that differences in desire and arousability may be linked to a dopamine receptor gene. There also is some evidence that there may be a genetic predisposition involved in dyspareunia. In separate studies, approximately 30% of women with dyspareunia reported having family members with the same problem. Genetic polymorphisms have been identified for PVD, and there appears to be a genetic susceptibility to inflammatory disorders (Burri, Cherkas, & Spector, 2009).

General Health and Medical Conditions

Data from large epidemiological studies consistently find associations between sexual problems and general health in both women and men (Laumann et al., 1999; Lewis et al., 2010). Women who report their health to be excellent are less likely to have a sexual dysfunction than women who rate their health lower. Lack of regular exercise has also been linked to sexual problems, as have emotional difficulties, stress, and substance abuse. There is ample theoretical and empirical support for the potential impact of a long list of general medical conditions on women's sexual function. On a very basic level, the mechanisms that govern the sexual response include the autonomic nervous system, the cardiovascular system, the endocrine system, and the musculoskeletal system. In addition, there is the psychological impact of disease on a woman's mood and self-concept. The available data indicate that when general medical conditions have an impact on sexual function in women they often do so quite generally, affecting desire, arousal, and orgasm simultaneously.

The major classes of medical/physical conditions that have an impact on desire, arousal, and orgasm problems in women are endocrinological disturbances, cardiovascular diseases, cancer, and sensory/mobility disabilities (see Table 4). In terms of endocrine-related problems, the aforementioned hypoestrogenism, androgen insufficiency, and hyperprolactinemia have all been linked to various aspects of sexual function in women and can occur as a function of congenital conditions (Turner syndrome), menopause (natural or surgical), adrenal disease, kidney disease, and iatrogenically produced problems. Diabetes mellitus has also been shown to reduce vaginal lubrication and orgasmic capacity, although the mechanism by which this occurs is not well understood. Much more is known about the link between cardiovascular disease and sexual function in men than in women, but blood flow is clearly a central component of the sexual response in women. Hypertension in women has indeed been associated with deficits in lubrication and in orgasmic frequency and intensity. Most types of cancers take a very high toll on the sexual function of women, especially those affecting the breasts and reproductive organs. This generalized and severe impact is believed to be related to both disease processes, treatments, and the understandable body image concerns of women who have undergone disfiguring surgeries. These effects often persist for long periods of time in cancer survivors (Brotto, Yule, & Breckon, 2010). Finally, conditions that impact peripheral sensitivity and mobility, such as multiple sclerosis and spinal cord injuries, can have dramatic effects on arousal and orgasm. Aside from these serious disabilities, there is now consistent evidence of sensory abnormalities in women with dyspareunia, both in the vulvar area and in nongenital sites, indicating abnormalities in central pain processing (Pukall et al., 2005).

Although a number of these diseases can impact lubrication and genital tissue so as to result in painful intercourse, there are other conditions that have specific associations with dyspareunia and vaginismus. Recurrent vaginal infections (mostly yeast), vaginal atrophy, genital trauma, and vaginal dermatoses have been linked to vulvar pain during intercourse. In the absence of longitudinal studies, causation can only be inferred. PVD is believed to be the most common cause of dyspareunia. Although the precise etiology of this condition remains unknown, it is characterized by hyperalgesia (extreme sensitivity) at the entry of the vagina (vulvar vestibule). This purported nerve dysfunction can render any contact (not just intercourse) with the vulvar vestibule excruciating. Another condition specifically linked to the sexual pain disorders is pelvic floor dysfunction. Painful intercourse can result from either hypertonic or hypotonic pelvic floor muscles. Most of these conditions can result in genital pain with intercourse; likewise, endometriosis, pelvic inflammatory disease, and various types of ovarian and other pelvic adhesions can produce deep pelvic pain during sexual activity.

Finally, urinary incontinence is a common problem for many women in perimenopause or postmenopause, with a significant impact on sexual function. Even if the incontinence is mild (commonly referred to as stress incontinence as it occurs only when stress is placed on the bladder or pelvic floor musculature, e.g., through coughing, running, laughing, or sneezing), the impact on sexual function can be quite severe. Women worry that they may secrete urine during penetration or orgasm, and their spontaneity can be curtailed by hygiene and odor concerns.

In summary, there are many general medical and physical conditions that, alone or in tandem with their treatment, constitute significant risk factors for sexual problems in women. Whether the mechanisms that impact sexual function are properties of a disease process, its treatment, or its psychological impact, clinicians need to assess for the involvement of medical factors. In clinical practice, general medical conditions are not reasons to refer out when a client presents with sexual dysfunction. Rather, they represent important components to be targeted by multidisciplinary treatments involving more than one health professional, when necessary.

Existence of a general medical condition does not preclude psychological treatment for sexual dysfunction

Medications

Prescription medications are common risk factors for sexual dysfunction in women (see Table 4). Selective serotonin reuptake inhibitors (SSRIs), antidepressants that increase circulating levels of serotonin, are among the most widely prescribed drugs, and they have been shown to have an inhibitory influence on desire, arousal, and orgasmic function (Rosen, Lane, & Menza, 1999). Dual-action antidepressant medications that inhibit the reuptake of serotonin as well as norepinephrine (SSNRIs) seem to produce lower levels of interference with arousal and desire (Meston et al., 2004). A number of antipsychotic medications have been shown to affect orgasmic function in women. Antiseizure drugs have been linked in the literature to less satisfying orgasms (Meston et al., 2004). Finally, there is some indication that experimenting with thyroid function medication may help women who are being treated pharmaceutically for thyroid irregularities and experiencing sexual problems as a consequence of this treatment.

Although the sexual side effects of these medications have been well-documented, they present a dilemma for the clinician. Sexual dysfunction is clearly undesirable, but it needs to be weighed against other potentially more serious consequences of the disorder for which these medications have been prescribed (e.g., major depression). Potential strategies include waiting for spontaneous remission of sexual side effects, choosing medications with minimal sexual side effects, reducing dosages, and the addition of secondary medications (antidotes) to counter the sexual function side effects (Ashton, 2007).

Sexual side effects of necessary medications can be targeted by cautious yet creative strategies on the part of the prescribing physician

Table 4
Classes of General Medical/Physical Conditions and Medications Associated With Sexual Dysfunctions in Women

Conditions

Endocrine-related
Menopause, prolactinemia, hypoestrogenism, androgen insufficiency, adrenal disease, kidney disease, diabetes, pituitary tumor

Cardiovascular
Hypertension, atherosclerosis, stroke

Cancer
Breast, reproductive organs, colon, rectal, and others

Sensory/mobility deficits
Multiple sclerosis, spinal cord injury

Genitourinary/pelvic
Provoked vestibulodynia, pelvic floor dysfunction, urinary incontinence, endometriosis, pelvic inflammatory disease, interstitial cystitis, pelvic and ovarian adhesions, cysts

Chronic pain

Medications

Antidepressants – Selective serotonin reuptake inhibitors
Antipsychotics
Antiseizure drugs
Estrogen inhibitors
Antihypertensives

Surgeries and Other Treatments

Bilateral oophorectomies
Simple hysterectomies
Radiotherapy
Chemotherapy

Surgery and Other Treatments

There are a number of surgeries and other systemic treatments that can significantly affect the sexual response of women (see Table 4). The surgery with the most obvious impact on sexual function is a bilateral oophorectomy. In the premenopausal woman this surgery will result in surgically induced menopause and, without hormone replacement therapy, the possibility of deficits in desire, lubrication, and orgasm, as well as dyspareunia. The data available on the impact of simple hysterectomies (in which the woman's ovaries are left intact) are less clear, but there is evidence that some women report the development of dysfunction as a result of the removal of the uterus alone. Genital procedures such as episiotomies have also been occasionally linked to dyspareunia, and the jury is still out on possible sexual function sequelae of cosmetic genital surgery. The most reasonable stance is for the clinician and client to consider any pelvic or genital surgery as potentially having an impact on sexual function.

Although dyspareunia often occurs with endometriosis (especially with cul-de-sac endometrial implants), the hormonal treatment of endometriosis has unfortunately been linked to HSDD. That is hardly a surprise as endometriosis is often treated medically with estrogen inhibitors. When estrogen/androgen production and circulation is interfered with, many women complain of significant and distressing decreases in sexual interest. Hysterectomies are also commonly performed in this population.

Cancer treatments can also negatively influence women's sexual responses. Breast cancer survivors commonly report multiple sexual difficulties linked to postsurgical body image concerns, as well as medical regimens that inhibit estrogen production. In cancers of the reproductive system, the negative impact of radical hysterectomies often cannot be addressed with hormone replacement therapy for fear of increasing the risk of certain malignancies. Radiotherapy of the pelvic region and certain types of chemotherapy can also shut down or impair ovarian function.

3.1.2   Psychological

There is no strong empirical evidence supporting the exclusive role of any particular psychological process or state in the etiology of sexual dysfunctions in women. What we have are (1) theoretical reasons to postulate that certain psychological states might predispose someone to sexual difficulties and (2) empirical evidence that certain cognitions and emotions consistently co-occur with sexual dysfunction. The determination of whether psychological factors are a cause or consequence of the development of sexual dysfunction is an important research endeavor. In terms of clinical practice, however, the distinction is academic. Whether depressive symptoms have triggered a reduction in sexual desire or whether a reduction in sexual desire has resulted over time in depressive symptoms, the clinician will have to target these symptoms equally directly and forcefully. It is not uncommon for psychological sequelae of sexual difficulties to actually become the greatest barriers to their resolution. As mentioned earlier, the factors that may have initiated a difficulty are not necessarily the ones that maintain it.

Thus, in the following sections, we will consider cognitive-affective correlates of sexual difficulties in women. Current science makes it impossible to ascertain their direct etiological involvement. We do have some evidence, however, that psychological factors can augment symptoms and interfere with the resolution of sexual problems.

Cognition
Although it is sometimes hard for both clients and clinicians to distinguish between cognitions and emotions, attempts to do so are at the heart of cognitive-behavioral therapy (CBT) and appear to be relatively effective in treatment. The identification of cognitions related to sexuality can be even more challenging. The self-report of general attitudes about sex is subject to fairly strong social desirability pressures, while identifying thoughts that occur during sex presents additional recall difficulties. Research has nonetheless investigated both and found some evidence of cognitions linked to sexual difficulties.

Negative Attitudes About Sexuality

Attitudes toward sexuality fluctuate and vary across generations, religions, and cultures. However, there is also within-group variability and that variability may have some relationship to sexual difficulties. Although sex therapists report that they now encounter far fewer cases than 3 decades ago of sexual dysfunction driven by negative sexual attitudes and misinformation, attitudes continue to play a role in certain cases.

For example, some women with low desire have been found to describe sex in negative ways with hints of displeasure, disgust, and devaluations of their more desiring partners (Sims & Meana, 2010). Conservative sexual values and religiosity have been linked (although not consistently) to various aspects of sexual function. In Portuguese samples, Nobre and Pinto-Gouveia (2006; 2008) reported that women with sexual dysfunctions endorsed more beliefs about menopause resulting in loss of sexual desire and about the inability of physically "unattractive women" to be sexually satisfied. Sexual conservatism and beliefs that sexual desire and pleasure are sinful were found more often in women with HSDD. SAD is by definition a dysfunction in which sex is viewed as negative and even disgusting. Negative sexual attitudes have also been found in women with dyspareunia (Meana, Binik, Khalife, & Cohen, 1997b). Of course, we often do not know whether the negative attitudes preceded the sexual difficulties or developed as a consequence. In either case, treatment would have to address negative attitudes about sex if they in fact exist.

Distraction

There is a significant body of work pointing to the role of distraction in sexual problems. As earlier reviewed, Barlow's model of sexual functioning posits that individuals with dysfunction shift their attention from erotic cues to internal concerns about the negative consequences of not performing. In this model, distraction and self-focused attention are counterproductive to an enjoyable sexual experience. Research on women with sexual dysfunction strongly supports the role of distraction. The distractors, however, may be quite different than they are in men.

Women with low desire have reported thinking about a variety of nonerotic cues during sex, mostly having to do with whatever was on their to-do list, from housekeeping to child care to professional concerns (Sims & Meana, 2010). This may be an indicator of the burden imposed by current lifestyles, wherein women are expected to be caretakers (of husband, children, and household) as well as income earners, or successful professionals. This type of general preoccupation is likely to have an impact primarily on desire, but also on arousal and orgasm. Distraction has even been linked to the sexual pain disorders, in laboratory research (Lykins, Meana, & Minimi, 2011).

It is clear that all aspects of the sexual response require attention to sensory input. To a certain extent, sexual arousal requires a cognitive withdrawal from the mundane concerns of daily life and a focus on sex or sexual fantasy. An inability to do that is likely to result in either an avoidance of sex or in a mechanical engagement that leaves both partners feeling empty, dissatisfied, and often angry. When sex is perceived as an obligation, a chore, or an interruption from supposedly more important things, sexual dysfunction has either already begun or is well on its way.

Generally speaking, women who report a large number of arousal contingencies (specific conditions under which they can get aroused) are essentially reporting a high degree of distractibility. If everything has to be "just so" in order for them to feel desire and become aroused, then cognitions are likely playing a significant interfering role in the sexual response. This type of high arousal contingency profile is not unusual in women with HSDD, FSAD, FOD, or even dyspareunia and vaginismus. In the case of the sexual pain disorders, pain is clearly the most significant distractor.

Self-Focus
In Barlow's research with men, self-focus was found to have a negative impact on sexual performance. Rather than attend to erotic cues provided by their partner, performance-anxious men tended to monitor their bodily changes (erections) and critically evaluate their physical arousal, leading mostly to negative results. Research with women, on the other hand, indicates that self-focus can be either positive or negative. It depends on how a woman feels about herself. If she evaluates herself to be sexy, the self-focus can be an arousal enhancer. It is thus the valence of self-focus during sexual activity that is the greater predictor of sexual enjoyment. When that valence is positive, self-consciousness can enhance desire and arousal. In a focus group study by Graham et al. (2004), women's feelings about their bodies were identified as important facilitators to arousal. In a related way, Trapnell, Meston, and Gorzalka (1997) found that a composite of three traits linked to dispositional nonpathological narcissism (flirtatious, seductive, and fashionable) significantly predicted sexual experience among men and women.

Positive self-focus may thus be a significant facilitator of desire. Women's sexuality may in fact have a significant component of autoeroticism (the extent to which one's appraisal of oneself as sexy is arousing in and of itself). A recent study reported that one third to one half of a sample of women reported arousal in contemplating themselves nude, wearing sexy lingerie or clothes, grooming, and imagining that others find them irresistible (Moser, 2009). These data suggest that interventions might be well-advised to attend to the enhancement of women's feelings about their own desirability rather than focus exclusively on partner-related factors. Unfortunately, many of the women who present with clinical problems have a decidedly negative valence to their self-focus during sex.

The way a woman feels about herself may be even more important to her sexual function than the way her partner feels about her

Body Image
There are a number of studies indicating that women are often distracted during sex by concerns about their appearance (e.g., Meana & Nunnink, 2006). Body dissatisfaction in women is now almost normative, and there is evidence that this negative self-image is interfering with sexual function. Referring back to Barlow's model, perhaps women consider their physical attractiveness to be a type of sexual performance. While men feel anxious about losing their erections, women may feel inadequate about their attractiveness failing them. Body image self-consciousness during sex is certainly very common (Wiederman, 2000). There is also some evidence that this negative body image may be relatively impervious to partner assurances.

In one study of women with HSDD, concerns about desirability featured prominently as attributions for their low desire, despite their husbands' compliments, desire, and repeated assertions of their attractiveness (Sims & Meana, 2010). A common report in that study was of worrying if the intercourse position they were engaging in was unflattering (e.g., worrying that if they were on top, their breasts would sag or their bellies would look bigger). Clinicians are advised to attend to how women feel about themselves, as this factor can be even more important than relational ones. A recent development of some concern is the increase in genital cosmetic surgery, evidence that social and other forces have now added genital image to women's already long list of bodily dissatisfactions. Genital self-image has been linked to sexual function, sexual behavior, and sexual and genital health care behavior in women (Herbenick et al., 2011).

Causal Attributions

Why a woman thinks she developed a sexual problem is important assessment and treatment planning information

Some women have no personal theories about why they are having sexual difficulties. They have no idea why they have little desire, problems becoming aroused or reaching orgasm, or why they have pain with sex. Other women, however, have developed theories about the etiology of their sexual dysfunction. Sometimes these are wholly self-generated and sometimes they are a combination of their own lay theory and a health care professional opinion. These theories are important to the clinician for at least three reasons: (1) they may be accurate and indicate a specific treatment strategy, (2) regardless of their accuracy, they may have causal force, and (3) they have been shown to be related to psychosocial adjustment.

Most of the empirical support for the impact of individuals' causal attributions for their disorders emanates from nonsexually related conditions. One study, however, found that women's casual attributions for pain during intercourse significantly predicted a number of important treatment variables. Meana, Binik, Khalife, and Cohen (1999) found that women who attributed their pain to psychological causes reported greater pain ratings, distress, sexual aversion, and interpersonal conflict, independently of gynecological test results.

Somatic Hypervigilance and Pain Catastrophization

There is now a fair amount of correlational evidence indicating that women with dyspareunia may attend more to somatic sensations than do women without pain. Young women with dyspareunia and women with PVD have been found in numerous studies to have an attentional bias toward bodily sensations and the potential risk therein (e.g., Granot, 2005; Meana & Lykins, 2009). Women with PVD also appear to be hypervigilant about genital pain in particular. The attentional focus on the pain is acute, and contrary to the other sexual dysfunctions, distraction from some of the sensations felt during sex may be a useful treatment strategy.

Pain catastrophization is also common in women with dyspareunia. The construct of pain catastrophization refers to an attentional bias for pain-related information, and it has been consistently linked to pain perception and disability in chronic pain patients. It is both a cognitive and an affective experience combining magnification, rumination, and helplessness (Sullivan, Lynch, & Clark, 2005). Women with vaginismus and dyspareunia commonly demonstrate high levels of pain catastrophization. The negative impact of this cognitive-affective style on pain perception and sexual experiences makes it a natural target for cognitive interventions. Again, there is no direct evidence that a predisposition to these cognitive styles results in the development of the sexual pain disorders, but there is evidence that these cognitions make matters worse.

Affect

As epidemiological surveys of community samples have shown, there are many women with low levels of desire, arousal, and orgasmic capacity who are not particularly distressed about their sexuality. This is important to keep in mind so that we do not pathologize individual differences in sexual expression or in the importance placed on sex. However, women who seek help are either personally distressed by their sexual function or they are distressed by its impact on a highly valued relationship. This negative affect can in turn further interfere with the sexual response.

Depression

There is consistent evidence for a strong negative correlation between depression and sexual desire, arousal, and orgasm in both men and women. In untreated major depression, sexual disinterest and arousal difficulties have been found in 50% of women (Kennedy, Dickens, Eisfeld, & Bagby, 1999). Women with a history of major depression manifest lower levels of arousal and pleasure, independent of current depressive symptoms (Cyranowski, Frank, Cherry, Huck, & Kupfer, 2004). Complicating the picture is the fact that many of the most effective antidepressants can also suppress sexual function.

Diagnosable mood disorders aside, women who complain about low sexual desire also demonstrate higher levels of negative affect, including mood lability, self-esteem concerns, and symptoms of anxiety (Hartmann, Philippsohn, Heiser, & Ruffer-Hesse, 2004). The sexual pain disorders have also been linked to depressive symptomatology (Meana et al., 1997b). Even very young women who experience dyspareunia at the start of their sexual lives report feelings of sadness and emotional dysregulation that they connect back to having pain with intercourse (Donaldson & Meana, 2011).

Anxiety and Fear

The relationship of anxiety to sexual function is more paradoxical than that of depression, at least experimentally. In some laboratory studies, the induction of anxiety has increased subjective and physical arousal in both functional and dysfunctional women (Meston & Bradford, 2007). However, in the self-report of clinical and community samples, anxiety is negatively linked to sexual function in women. Because of the distracting nature of anxiety, with its common list of worries and preoccupations, it is intuitive that it would interfere with desire, arousal, and orgasm, all of which require focus on erotic thoughts, stimuli, and sensations. In the case of the sexual pain disorders, the anxiety appears to play a particularly central role.

Anxiety is easily the emotional state most closely associated with sexual dysfunction

Women with PVD have demonstrated higher levels of state and trait anxiety than nondysfunction controls (Payne, Binik, Amsel, & Khalife, 2005). Regardless of whether anxious women are more likely to develop sexual pain disorders, it is certainly understandable why the anticipation of pain might create anxiety. Even if the anxiety is specific to the impending experience of pain with penetration, it is also likely to be interfering with arousal which in turn will make the penetration even more uncomfortable. It is a classic vicious cycle. Within samples of women with dyspareunia, differences in anxiety have been linked to the perception of pain, the enjoyment of sexual interactions, and the avoidance of sex.

In a recent study, young women with dyspareunia also scored higher than controls on anxiety sensitivity, which is a tendency to interpret anxiety-related symptoms (e.g., increased heart rate, perspiration, or muscle tension) as portents of severe physical, social, or psychological outcomes (Meana & Lykins, 2009). As previously discussed, pain catastrophization in part captures this strong affective reaction and its sequelae. In women with vaginismus, this anxiety reaches phobic levels and can best be described as all-out fear. The fear leads to an extreme avoidant pattern of behavior whereby sexual intercourse is no longer attempted and gynecological examinations are considered to be impossible.

Sexual Traumatization

Although not all women who have experienced childhood sexual abuse (CSA) develop sexual problems as adults, a significant number do. They generally have a higher prevalence of desire, arousal, and orgasm dysfunctions than women with no such experiences (Leonard & Follette, 2002). Even when the sexual difficulties do not rise to the level of a diagnosable dysfunction, their levels of satisfaction with sex tend to be lower. In addition, a number of the sexual symptoms reported by these women may not fit neatly into DSM categories, but nonetheless be distressing and interfering. These include shame and guilt about their sexual responses (Hall, 2007). Cognitive-affective processes that might mediate the relationship between CSA and adult sexual functioning in women are a negative view of sexuality and a negative sense of self (Meston & Heiman, 2000). In women with a history of CSA, sympathetic nervous system activation does not facilitate physiological arousal as it can in women without such histories (Rellini & Meston, 2006). This may be due in part to a pairing of these sensations with traumatic memories. Sexual assault occurring during adulthood (rape or attempted rape) is also associated with sexual difficulties in women at all stages of the sexual response.

Although some studies have not found a link between lifetime sexual abuse (SA) and the sexual pain disorders (Meana et al., 1997b), there is increasing evidence that women with a history of SA are indeed overrepresented in clinical and community samples of women with dyspareunia and vaginismus. Women presenting with dyspareunia have been found to be 2.7 times more likely to have experienced CSA (Latthe, Mignini, Gray, Hills, & Khan, 2006), and women with vulvar pain were 6.5 times more likely to report severe sexual abuse than no-pain controls. In terms of vaginismus, one study found women with this condition to be twice as likely to have experienced what the authors termed "sexual interference" (Reissing, Binik, Khalife, Cohen, & Amsel, 2003).

Personality

The research linking personality and sexual dysfunction in women is scarce and can be conceptually questionable depending on the definition of constructs and interpretation of results. Although personality generally refers to characteristic behavioral and cognitive-affective patterns, it is hard to know in the case of sexual dysfunction, the extent to which said patterns preceded the dysfunction or developed as a function of it. This is particularly true when the sexual dysfunction is long-standing. The danger inherent in the use of the construct of personality is that it generally implies an inherent quality of the individual, divorced from situational stressors.

In any case, women with sexual dysfunctions, low sexual satisfaction, and general sexual maladjustment generally have higher neuroticism scores than norms or controls (e.g., Granot, 2005; Meana & Lykins, 2009). Neuroticism basically amalgamates several dimensions of negative affect and may indicate a general unhappiness that could be situational or dispositional. Extraversion scores are lower in women with diagnosable sexual dysfunction at all stages of the sexual response and with sexual pain. Overall, it seems that some women with sexual dysfunction are characterized by higher levels of negative affect as well as interpersonal and social discomfort. Women with sexual pain disorders may also tend toward a cognitive style marked by anxious thoughts that focus on bodily symptoms and toward catastrophization of these symptoms. Only treatment outcome studies will be able to elucidate if these are trait or state characteristics. In the chronic pain literature, pain treatment has been shown to improve "personality" scores. Further research will indicate whether the same is true in the case of women's sexual dysfunctions.

Distinguishing a personality trait from a state of distress related to sexual dysfunction can be difficult

3.1.3 Social

Couple Relationship

The quality of a couple's relationship seems to be the most obvious risk factor for sexual dysfunction. Certainly it is the one that mental health clinicians have most often targeted for intervention. After all, sexual function difficulties play out primarily in a relational context. If the sexual difficulty does not arise from the relationship itself, it is likely affecting it, as it can significantly diminish the couple's pleasure and intimacy. The positive association between sexual satisfaction and relationship quality has been found in many studies (e.g., Sprecher & Cate, 2004). Thus, assessing the couple's relationship dynamics (sexual or otherwise) is a key component of most interventions for sexual dysfunction. It is important to remember, however, that there are many well-adjusted couples who experience sexual problems. Clinicians who persist with a relational treatment strategy when relationship problems are not at the heart of the difficulty can do damage.

Relationship Duration

The data on relationship duration and sexual drive are pretty clear. Sexual desire and arousal generally appear to be highest at the beginning of the relationship and decline over time. This course may be particularly pronounced for women (Meana, 2010). Although couples can enjoy satisfying sex for the length of their relationship, it can be helpful for both clinicians and clients to keep in mind that some decrease is normative. In one study of married women with HSDD, the institutionalization of the relationship, overfamiliarity, and the desexualization of roles, which can happen as a function of routine married

Keeping passion alive in long-term relationships generally requires special attention

life and parenting, were invoked as barriers to sexual desire (Sims & Meana, 2010). Long-term relationships, even good ones, can be hard on passion. Knowing that, and targeting it, can be helpful.

Discrepancies in Desire

One of the most common problems in couples presenting with sexual difficulties is discrepancies in desire or arousability (Clement, 2002). Most clinicians report that, in heterosexual couples, the woman is more commonly the lower desire partner. This is hardly surprising considering women's significantly higher rates of HSDD. The person with the lower desire tends to be the one who gets the diagnosis, but it is important to determine whether there really is a desire deficit linked to possibly important biogenesis or psychogenesis or whether it is simply a desire discrepancy between partners. The treatment can vary significantly, contingent on this determination. Original discrepancies in desire can, however, develop into sexual dysfunctions (1) if the lower desire partner experiences years of badgering that can result in mild to moderate sexual aversion or (2) if the higher desire partner reacts to the perceived rejection with a loss of sexual desire or arousability of his or her own. Some of these relationships can end up being sexless.

Partner Sexual Dysfunction

One person's sexual dysfunction can give rise to dysfunction in his/her partner

The presence of a sexual dysfunction in the partner can also be a significant risk factor. In large cross-national representative samples of heterosexual women, low desire, lubrication problems, orgasm difficulty, and dyspareunia have all been consistently and strongly related to perceived erectile dysfunction in the male partner. Lubrication and orgasm problems have also been linked to perceived delayed and premature ejaculation in partners (Jiann, Su, Yu, & Huang, 2009). It is easy to hypothesize numerous ways in which a sexual difficulty in one partner can engender a parallel difficulty in the other. Erectile dysfunction can be perceived by women as lack of desire or attraction to them. It can also result in stress-filled attempts at penetration that either happen before the woman is adequately aroused or after her arousal has abated. Premature ejaculation can also result in insufficient stimulation for the woman, and delayed ejaculation can result in the irritation of vulvar and vaginal tissue as a function of overly forceful or lengthy thrusting. Dysfunction in the partner is thus an important assessment component and treatment indicator as it appears to be closely linked to sexual dysfunction in the woman.

Relationship/Marital Satisfaction

A multitude of studies have reported an association between sexual desire in women and relationship quality. Good relationship quality (e.g., marital satisfaction, marital happiness, and intimacy) has been linked to more frequent sexual desire or lower desire discrepancy between partners. Marital satisfaction has been linked to higher arousability and orgasm frequency. Conversely, couples reporting sexual problems report less relationship satisfaction, more conflict, and less skillful communication. The list of negative relationship dynamics linked to sexual problems is long and includes frequent arguments, anger, sexual communication difficulties, less closeness, less intimacy, fewer feelings of love, and hostility.

There is less empirical evidence for the link between relationship discord and the sexual pain disorders than for other sexual dysfunctions (Davis & Reissing, 2007). Yet it is hard to imagine that there would not be negative effects of sexual pain on dyadic relationships. Qualitative research certainly points in that direction, with young women reporting significant relationship conflict as a function of their difficulties with penetration (Donaldson & Meana, 2011). Perhaps clinical observations and research with partnered women who have pain with intercourse obfuscate the impact of these disorders on those women whose relationships did not survive the sexual dysfunction. Hostility in the partner has in fact been found to be related to pain intensity in women with PVD (Desrosiers et al., 2008). Pain ratings in women with dyspareunia have also been linked to marital adjustment (Meana, Binik, Khalife, & Cohen, 1998).

Partner Solicitousness
Specifically in relation to dyspareunia, partner solicitousness has been found to predict pain intensity (Desrosiers et al., 2008). Solicitousness refers to a reactive pattern characterized by demonstrations of sympathy, attention, and support for the person with an illness or with chronic pain. Although this behavioral-emotive pattern in a partner sounds positive and is well-intentioned, it may in fact encourage illness behavior and pain catastrophization. This is of clinical significance as partner responses to pain may be important intervention targets. Thus far, the evidence indicates that there is a happy medium between negative reactions and overly empathic ones.

Family of Origin
Although there is scant research investigating the relationship of family of origin variables to sexuality (other than those related to CSA), a good part of sex education comes from families, either explicitly or implicitly. Families differ in their openness about sexual matters, in their sex positivity, and in the ways in which parents model the dynamics of intimate, sexual relationships. Research with adolescents indicates that parents remain important sources of sexual information, and individual differences in sexual attitudes have been linked to parental strictness about sexual matters (Fisher, Byrne, White, & Kelley, 1988).

Families thus, advertently and inadvertently, provide scripts about sexuality. Often clients will state that their families did not talk about sex or that their parents rarely demonstrated signs of having a romantic, sexual relationship. Clients often do not realize that this type of sexual silence is also a strong communicator of sexual values. Because of the sexual double standard adopted by many families, women's sexuality may be at higher risk for negative family-of-origin influences. The current weight of evidence indicates that parental and family environments have a stronger effect on the sexual behavior of daughters than on that of sons (Baumeister, 2000). Although there is no hard evidence linking specific family environments to sexual dysfunction, developmental factors are possible contributors to sexual difficulties in women. Research does show that a positive sexual self-schema (one's consideration of oneself as a sexual being) in women is related to higher arousability, more positive attitudes about sex, and longer lasting sexual relationships (Andersen

& Cyranowski, 1994). Complicating matters further, each partner may enter their relationship with different and sometimes conflicting family-of-origin-influenced sexual scripts.

Sociocultural

The mainstream training of clinical psychologists tends to be focused on individual factors. Consequently, clinicians sometimes fail to give appropriate weight to the social forces that can contribute to maladaptive behaviors and negative cognitions and emotions. Yet, throughout our life span we are bombarded with messages, explicit and implicit, about the appropriate sexual roles of men and women, about when (age and timing) and what type of sexual experience is acceptable (activities, partners, and contexts), and about how sexual experiences should unfold (a normative sequence of events). These are sexual scripts. The extent to which these scripts conform or magnify biological predispositions or evolutionarily adaptive functions is beyond the scope of this book. Regardless, theoretical reasoning and empirical research indicate that these scripts can have a damaging impact on sexual function and relationships (McCormick, 2010).

The Sexual Double Standard

The sexual double-standard script wherein men and women are judged differently for the same sexual behavior is still alive and well in the 21st century. Men are expected to be sexually aggressive and consistent performers, and women are expected to be less interested and more submissive receivers of male desire. This persistent sexual double standard can result in feelings of inadequacy and shame for both men and women. The general suppression of authentic female sexual expression and silencing of adolescent girls' sexual desire has been well documented (Tolman, 2002). Alternately, the constant comparison with men's desire as if it were the gold standard can leave women feeling insufficiently sexual. Historically, it has been hard for women to know how much sexual desire is just right. If you have too little you are frigid; too much and you are a "nymphomaniac." There appears to be a pretty narrow range of acceptable sexual desire for women, at least according to dominant sexual scripts.

Ageism

Most societies have fairly rigid scripts about age and sexuality. Elderly sex is practically considered an oxymoron, despite data indicating that many older adults continue to consider sex an important quality-of-life component. Oppenheimer (2002) identified three themes of this nearly universal sexual script about older adults: desire for discretion (it is better not to talk about sex and the elderly); disgust and abhorrence; and focus on the deterioration of sexual organs rather than on the affection, closeness, and companionship aspects of sexual activity.

The age-appropriate script also generally has a sexual double standard built into it. It is particularly restrictive of women, who are divested of their status as sexual beings well before men are. The societal desexualization of women as young as 45 can have a significant impact on women's sexual self-schema. If society no longer relates to you as desirable, it becomes hard for you to do so yourself. It may also have an impact on your partner's feelings. These insidious societal messages can seep into the most personal of moments.

Adherence to normative beliefs about age-appropriate sexuality has been linked to sexual dysfunction in women. In one study, women with a sexual dysfunction endorsed more age-related beliefs than women without sexual complaints (Nobre & Pinto-Gouveia, 2006). They were more likely to endorse beliefs such as "after menopause, women lose their sexual desire." Society continues to communicate that sexual activity among elderly adults is somehow inappropriate and even disgusting, especially for women. It would thus not be surprising for these forceful and ubiquitous messages to affect the lives of clients. Research shows that even some health professionals working with older adults subscribe to these prejudices (Lai & Hynie, 2011).

Coitus Priority

Another normative sexual script that can be damaging to sexual function is the belief that only penile-vaginal intercourse constitutes sex. Even among recent studies of young men and women on college campuses, intercourse is considered to be sex more often than other equally intimate activities, such as fellatio or cunnilingus. This belief demotes all other types of sexual activity as secondary to the "main event" and poses undue pressure on both men and women. Men are required to be sufficiently erect, and women are expected to be orgasmic with intercourse. The rest of what goes on in a complex sexual encounter is deemed less important.

Clearly, the coitus priority theme does no justice to the multiple and multifaceted pleasures that a sexual encounter can provide. But this script can be particularly damaging to women, as the majority of women require clitoral stimulation to achieve orgasm, over and above that provided by intercourse alone. A couple's assessment of their sexual function can be negatively affected by this script. Women and their partners may believe that the woman has FOD when all she needs is additional stimulation. Similarly, a man may believe that he is not erect for long enough to please his partner, when all she really needs is an alternate strategy.

The Spontaneity Script

An additional very common sexual script creates the expectation that sex should happen much like spontaneous combustion. Although this may appear to happen at the beginning of relationships, it is a rarer occurrence in long-term relationships, when partners are coping with habituation and multiple demands on their time, including professional and parenting ones. Rigidly adhering to an expectation of spontaneity in sexual interactions can leave couples feeling as if they have "lost that loving feeling." This may be particularly problematic for women, whose sexual desire has been hypothesized to be more responsive (rather than spontaneous) in nature. A woman or her partner rigidly adhering to the spontaneity script may end up pathologizing what in fact are normal desire levels. In addition, interventions designed to reignite desire are undoubtedly not going to feel spontaneous. Challenging this unrealistic and paradoxically tyrannical (*be spontaneous, now!*) sexual script component can do wonders for a couple's sex life.

The Sexless Motherhood Script

Waiting for spontaneous sex can result in no sex at all

Classical psychoanalysis referred to a Madonna–whore complex whereby certain men seemed incapable of combining both love and lust for the same woman, as if these emotions were incompatible. Not surprisingly, women also have a hard time seeing themselves fulfilling the dual roles of lover and mother. This is perhaps most obvious in mothers with children still at home. Parenting can have a dampening effect on the sexual lives of couples for very practical reasons, especially when the children are young. The loss of privacy, concerns about exposing children to the sexual component of the couple's relationship, overscheduling, and fatigue are just some of the aspects of parenting that can interfere with a couple's sex life. However, some women also seem to have a harder time seeing themselves as sexual beings once they enter motherhood. In one study of women with acquired HSDD, many attributed their loss of desire to the incompatibility of their roles as mothers and wives (Sims & Meana, 2010). Although not much research has been conducted on this topic, the sentiment is encountered in clinical settings quite often.

Socioeconomic Disadvantage and Lifestyle Stress

Epidemiological studies consistently find a link between socioeconomic status and sexual dysfunction in both men and women. In the largest US study conducted, women who had graduated from college were half as likely to experience low sexual desire, problems achieving orgasm, and sexual pain, as women who had not completed high school. Lower income levels, and especially deterioration in income level, are also associated with sexual dysfunction in women. Note the difference in sexual complaints between women living below the poverty line versus women with family incomes six times or more that level: sexual pain, 16.2% versus 11.4%; sex not pleasurable, 23.3 % versus 17.3%; unable to achieve orgasm, 27.4% versus 20.8%; lacked interest in sex, 39.7% versus 27.5%. The only sexual complaint more common in financially well-off women in that study was trouble with lubrication (Laumann, Paik, & Rosen, 1999). One can reasonably surmise that the stress of living in disadvantaged conditions interferes significantly with sexual function and satisfaction. Although clinicians are rarely in a position to have an impact on the socioeconomic conditions of their clients, an awareness of how these factors may be contributing to the problem can be helpful in treatment planning and support.

Stress and sex are not good bedfellows

Another type of socially engineered stress that can affect the sexual lives of women is multiple demands on their time. Some of the advances that have been made in terms of workplace gender equality over the past 5 decades may have paradoxically also increased the work burden on women. Their mass entry into the workforce has not been accompanied by a commensurate relief from their duties as housekeepers, parents, and caregivers to their own elderly parents. Research consistently shows that in full-time working couples, women continue to carry a larger proportion of the housekeeping, child, and family care burden. These circumstances can interfere with women's sex lives significantly. Married women with HSDD have reported that their multiple responsibilities make it difficult to feel in the mood for sex. For some, sex becomes another chore or obligation to add to their already too long to-do list (Sims & Meana, 2010).

4

Treatment

4.1   Methods of Treatment

Psychological interventions for sexual dysfunction have an interesting empirical validation history. Masters and Johnson (1970) cited very low "failure" rates (e.g., 0% for vaginismus and 22.8% for secondary orgasmic dysfunction in women) in their treatment outcome studies with more than 500 couples. They appeared to herald an era of relatively quick and successful resolution to sexual problems. Unfortunately, the future did not bear this out. After a flurry of studies in the subsequent decade, psychological treatment outcome research for sexual dysfunction (sex therapy) came to a near halt. In addition, the early success rates were never close to being replicated. Today, there are only a handful of randomized controlled trials (RCTs) of nonpharmaceutical treatment outcomes for sexual dysfunction in women. They all report modest efficacy, mostly leave the question of prognostic indicators unanswered, and struggle with the operationalization of treatment success.

The possible reasons for the paucity of psychological treatment outcome studies for sex therapy are legion and beyond the scope of this book. Research funding, though, is probably at the top of the list. Consider the contrasting explosion of sexual dysfunction assessment research. As pharmaceutical companies raced to find agents that could target sexual difficulties, assessment tools to evaluate the outcome of pharmaceutical clinical trials proliferated. This has generally been a positive development. Psychometrically sound outcome assessment tools are an essential component of the empirical validation of treatments, and we now have a bevy of these. The focus on function rather than satisfaction in some of these measures arguably fails to capture the complexity of the sexual experience, but they are nonetheless a welcome addition to the assessment arsenal. Now we just need the RCTs on psychological interventions for sexual dysfunction.

Psychological treatment outcome research for sexual dysfunctions has lagged far behind research on the development of psychometrically sound assessment tools

Despite the unfortunate paucity of RCTs in the area of women's sexual dysfunction, there is a collective body of knowledge that points in certain treatment directions. Sound theory, a handful of RCTs, a larger number of uncontrolled studies, and a wealth of clinical knowledge are the bases for today's version of evidence-based treatment. As Kazdin (2008) states, "Our field would profit enormously from codifying the experiences of clinicians in practice so that the information is accumulated and can be drawn on to generate and test hypotheses" (p. 155).

The contribution of clinical experience to the following pages is in part a consequence of the lack of RCTs. Although it would clearly be ideal to test all of the treatment recommendations in this book empirically, neither clients nor clinicians can wait for that complex enterprise to be completed. Clients are in distress in the present. We can wait for the perfectly designed study, or we can try some of the following theoretically well-grounded and, to varying extents, evidence-based interventions.

As outlined in previous sections, the female sexual dysfunctions are highly comorbid and share many risk factors, dysfunction-maintaining factors, and treatment indicators. To avoid redundancy, the following two sections will first cover general treatment guidelines and provide a general template for a recommended course and content of therapy likely to be applicable to all of the female sexual dysfunctions. This will be followed by separate sections outlining dysfunction-specific assessment and interventions that can be incorporated into the general template. Flexibility is, of course, recommended, as every client, problem, and clinician is different, and there is no established empirical validation for each of the various combinations of interventions presented.

4.1.1   General Assessment and Treatment Guidelines

Clinician Self-Efficacy and Comfort

Every subdiscipline stakes a justified claim to expert or in-depth knowledge about a specific area. Every subdiscipline is also naturally invested in protecting its professional boundaries. The distinctions, however, can be overstated. There are clinical psychologists who specialize in anxiety disorders, but most clinical psychologists will tell you that they can treat anxiety. Likewise, clinical psychologists who do not consider themselves sex therapists or specialists in sexuality can also be effective in helping many clients overcome or manage sexual difficulties.

Most of the principles and practices of sex therapy are very similar to the cognitive-behavioral interventions used to help clients manage other problems. Treating a sexual problem may require extra research about the client's particular dilemma, but this type of continuing education is something most practicing psychologists engage in when they encounter other issues that are not sexual in nature. There is no doubt that clinicians who specialize in sexu-

---

Disadvantages of Referring a Client Out When They Present With a Sexual Problem

The automatic referral out can be experienced as dismissive.

The probability that the client will act on that second referral may be low.

The stigma associated with a sex therapist consultation may be greater than that with a general psychologist.

Sex therapy is not likely to be covered to the same extent by health insurance.

Outside of large urban centers, sex therapists may be hard to find.

If the client is an existing one, the already obtained in-depth knowledge of the client will be helpful in understanding the dynamics of the sexual problem. The client will not have to start from scratch with a new therapist.

ality and see only sex therapy cases will be more knowledgeable and have more information at their fingertips. On the other hand, referring a client out because they have revealed a sexual dysfunction has some real disadvantages (see Summary Box). Referring out is wise when the presenting problem exceeds therapist competence, but sexuality should arguably be within every clinician's competence, considering that it is an integral part of virtually every client's life.

The toughest challenge in taking the step to treat sexual dysfunction is not the acquisition of knowledge about sexual dysfunction or about specific sex therapy interventions, but rather being comfortable discussing and addressing sexual concerns. The taboo surrounding sexuality affects therapists as much as it affects clients. When therapists are new to the area of sexuality, they struggle with a number of concerns (see Summary Box, below). These are natural and are usually overcome through exposure and experience. The fact is that most clients will be very grateful to be asked about sexuality and very relieved to be able to talk about it with a professional. Of course, if a therapist is unable to overcome their discomfort addressing sexual issues, despite concerted attempts, then the client should be referred out. Being at ease addressing sexual issues is the first and most important skill for the clinician. The interventions, as will be demonstrated, are well within the reach of the generalist clinical psychologist.

> **The best way to become comfortable talking with clients about sexual issues is to do it when indicated. The attempt will be met with relief and gratitude**

Common Therapist Concerns and Worries About Assessing and Treating Sexual Difficulties

Will I sound or look awkward or embarrassed asking questions about sexuality?

Will it embarrass my client?

How much detail do I ask for?

What if the client feels that my questions are gratuitous or curious?

Will I know what to ask about?

What if they present with sexual behavior I did not even know existed?

How will I know what is amenable to treatment and what is not when the line between function and dysfunction is so blurry?

I do not have perfect sex either. Who am I to treat people who are dissatisfied with their sex lives?

Multisystem/Multidisciplinary Assessment

In concert with the biopsychosocial framework, the assessment of the client's complaint needs to be multidisciplinary, unless otherwise indicated. The initial stance is that physiological, psychological, and socio-cultural-relational factors are all potentially influencing the sexual symptoms presented. In certain cases, the client's presentation will rule out one or more of these three categories as significant etiologically, but the problem may still be playing out on all dimensions. For example, a woman presenting with no sexual desire may claim that it has nothing to do with her husband, whom she finds attractive and gets along with. That does not mean the relationship is not being affected or that there is not some dynamic in the relationship that may be interfering with a resolution to the problem.

Remaining open to the possibility that client attributions for their dysfunction can be faulty is important, as clients can be strongly influenced by normative explanations for why things go wrong sexually (e.g., I have no desire because it is inappropriate for a woman of my age to be enthusiastic about sexuality). On the other hand, even grossly inaccurate client attributions can have powerful causal force and are always important to take into account when assessing and planning treatments. A good assessment rule of thumb is to conduct a comprehensive assessment of all clients, regardless of the presentation. More often than not, the assessment will unveil areas well outside the client's initial conceptualization that are fertile for intervention. The worst that can come out of a comprehensive assessment is the confirmation of areas that do not need to be targeted.

The challenge of a multisystem/multidisciplinary assessment can be one of resources and/or client willingness. It is not necessary to send every woman presenting with low desire to an endocrinologist. It is not always practical either. It entails an expense, and sometimes clients do not want to investigate or reinvestigate certain avenues (e.g., I know my low desire is associated with my menopause but I refuse hormone replacement therapy, so I don't want to be checked for that). The recommendation is simply that the assessment philosophy be one that considers possible interference on sexual function from various sources.

Treatment-Integrated Assessment

A multisystem/multidisciplinary conceptualization of sexual problems places a significant burden on assessment, as it broadens the number of areas to be considered. Treatment, however, cannot wait for the comprehensive assessment of all possible contributors to the problem. The patient's distress requires immediate intervention. The initial assessment thus provides a snapshot of the problem, usually with some relatively strong leads on the more problematic dimensions. As the treatment plan targets these initial leads, further assessment has to be integrated throughout the treatment for at least three important reasons: (1) Certain more sensitive issues may not be uncovered at the initial intake because their disclosure requires a level of trust and rapport that has not yet been established; (2) The treatment itself is likely to raise issues that were not evident at intake either for the client or for the clinician; and (3) Treatment-integrated assessment is central to treatment outcome monitoring and redirection, if necessary.

Concurrent Multidisciplinary Treatment

Multidisciplinary assessment may indicate multidisciplinary treatment, as determined by the results of the evaluation. If such is the case, the timing of the treatments is also important. As our understanding of physiological factors in the development of sexual dysfunction has grown, the treatment of sexual problems has incorporated other health professionals (e.g., urologists, gynecologists, physical therapists, and endocrinologists). When an organic etiology is suspected, clients have generally been referred to an appropriate physician who can treat the medical problem. The patient might then be referred back, if the medical/surgical treatment does not succeed. The strength of this approach has been its multidisciplinary nature, but the sequential course of these referrals ignores the fact that multiple factors are often working simultaneously to maintain the dysfunction. This type of sequential multidisciplinary treatment all but ignores these important interactions. The ideal is thus a concurrent multidisciplinary approach wherein there is a coordinated treatment effort by as many health professionals as indicated. This is no different from how we treat depression or anxiety. When we refer clients out for psychotropic medication, we do not generally terminate therapy and ask them to come back only if the antidepressant regimen does not work.

Not every woman who presents with a sexual problem will need to be followed by a gynecologist or other health care professional. As a matter of fact, most will not be. Issues related to mood, self-concept, sexual history, and relationships will predominate. However, it is a good idea to develop a list of other local health professionals who can become part of the treatment team if the problem requires intervention on various dimensions.

When more than one health professional is necessary to treat a sexual problem, they should work concurrently as a team

Treating Individuals and Couples

The majority of women presenting with a sexual dysfunction are partnered. Sometimes the couple will present for therapy, and sometimes the woman will present alone. Because of the primacy of the relationship in both the mechanical and emotional aspects of sex, it is recommended that assessment and treatment involve both partners as much as possible. It is helpful to tell clients that every sexual problem is actually a couple problem. This works to depathologize the client and it co-opts the partner into the treatment effort. Involving the partner is also practically important so as to effectively assess and intervene at many levels, including the partner's own possible dysfunction or misinformation, as well as mutual skills building, communication, behavioral activation, stimulus control, and emotional support. There can be resistance to partner involvement on the part of both women and their partners if they have conceptualized the problem as belonging to the presenting woman exclusively. This is important diagnostic information. Resistance can also emanate from not wanting to involve a new partner for fear of losing them or scaring them off. Although the preferred mode of treatment is couples therapy, clinicians also have to be flexible and work individually with women when the preferred alternative is, for some reason, not possible.

Even within a couple-focused treatment, there may also be instances in which individual sessions are helpful. For example, it may be preferable to teach a woman how to practice stimulating herself to orgasm or how to perform vaginal dilatation, without her partner being present. Or the client may want to explore some past trauma privately. Alternating between individual sessions and couple sessions requires some skill and rule setting regarding an agreed-upon management of secrets with appropriate informed consent. However, this approach can accelerate progress and keep the partner invested by involving him/her only in sessions that will engage them completely.

The sexual problem of either partner is really the sexual problem of both

If the woman presenting with sexual dysfunction is single, she is most commonly presenting with a sexual problem that she believes has either contributed to the dissolution of a relationship or is interfering with her finding or progressing in one. Vaginismus and sexual aversion are two of the more obvious cases in point. Although the lack of a partner can complicate treatment to the extent that practice within the couple context is not possible, a number of interventions can be quite effectively administered to an individual woman. The ultimate test of treatment efficacy in these cases is obviously delayed until the woman engages in partnered sexual activity.

4.1.2 Generic Therapy Template

Treatment consists of cognitive restructuring, emotional regulation, stimulus control and behavioral activation, and relationship skills-building

The following template describes three generic stages in the assessment and treatment of sexual dysfunction in women: an initial stage, a second stage that forms the core of the therapy, and a third stage focused on the consolidation of gains and relapse prevention. Each stage consists of assessment and treatment elements that have been found useful across the female sexual dysfunctions. In fact, the vast majority of psychological interventions in the sexual dysfunction literature are not dysfunction-specific (Binik & Meana, 2009). These include (1) cognitive restructuring, (2) emotional regulation, (3) stimulus control and behavioral activation, and (4) relationship skills building. Techniques that have been developed for specific sexual dysfunctions will be covered after the generic template is presented, but almost all fall into one of the above four categories.

Note that these categories of interventions emanate from the generalist's arsenal of interventions and are well within the knowledge base of most clinicians. The novelty is in their application to the complex set of factors that either give rise to sexual dysfunction or maintain it. For brevity's sake, the following three stages and their components assume the presence of a couple, but most are easily adaptable to individuals.

The generic therapy template can be used as a general treatment planning map for all female sexual dysfunctions. Depending on the specifics of the presenting case, the therapist can select from the general interventions in the template. These interventions have been empirically validated to varying degrees in the treatment of sexual and other problems. Following a consideration of the generic template, the therapist can then refer to the dysfunction-specific interventions that follow and add these to the treatment plan as appropriate.

Stage 1: Assess, Educate, Set Goals, Reduce Distress

The overriding goal of the initial stage of therapy involves gaining and providing as much understanding about the problem as possible, deciding on a course of action, and reducing distress. One way of typifying this stage is as a journey from confusion to clarity. A clear take on the problem is often experienced as therapeutic, in and of itself, and is clearly requisite for an effective treatment plan. Sometimes, achieving clarity is painstaking, as the major factors driving or maintaining the sexual difficulty can be well hidden from the clinician and from the client herself. It is not unusual for the central problem to be discovered only once a treatment plan is initiated to target an entirely different problem.

Assessment of the Sexual Problem

Clinical interview. There is currently no widely used, validated, standardized interview for the sexual dysfunctions such as exist for other DSM disorders. The clinical interview thus remains the main assessment technique with which to assess and diagnose sexual dysfunctions. Clinical interview guidelines have been proposed by multiple authors, and there is much overlap among the iterations (e.g., Meana, Binik, & Thaler, 2008). The initial assessment of the sexual problem should ideally consist of the client's (and her partner's) open-ended description of, and attributions for, the problem. The clinician may then ask more specific questions about the extent of the problem and the conditions under which it occurs. Appendices 2 and 3 provide a reasonable set of initial assessment questions and areas to investigate, regardless of the specific dysfunction the client presents with. They essentially cover the risk factors for sexual dysfunction.

Questionnaire measures. There are standardized questionnaire measures of general sexual function and couple adjustment that can be helpful in the initial assessment, as well as to monitor treatment progress. Table 5 provides a

Table 5
Measures of Global Sexual Function/Satisfaction and Relationship Adjustment

Measure	Reference
For Use With Women, Men, and Couples	
Derogatis Interview for Sexual Functioning (DISF/DISF-SR)	Derogatis (1997)
Golombok-Rust Inventory of Sexual Satisfaction (GRISS)	Rust & Golombok (1986)
Index of Sexual Satisfaction (ISS)	Hudson et al. (1981)
Sexual Interaction Inventory (SII)	LoPiccolo & Steger (1974)
Dyadic Adjustment Scale (DAS)	Spanier (1976)
For Use With Women	
Female Sexual Function Index (FSFI)	Rosen et al. (2000)
McCoy Female Sexuality Questionnaire (MFSQ)	McCoy & Matyas (1998)
Sexual Function Questionnaire (SFQ)	Quirk et al. (2002)
Brief Index of Sexual Functioning for Women (BISF-W)	Taylor et al. (1994)
Female Sexual Distress Scale (FSDS)	Derogatis et al. (2002)
Sexual Satisfaction Scale for Women (SSS-W)	Meston & Trapnell (2005)
For Use With Men	
Sexual Health Inventory for Men (SHIM/IIEF-5)	Rosen et al. (1999)
International Index of Erectile Function (IIEF)	Rosen et al. (2002)
Male Sexual Health Questionnaire (MSHQ) (specific to aging men)	Rosen, Catania et al. (2004)

list of these general sexual and couple adjustment measures. Some of these are specific to women, some to men, and some are designed to assess couple functioning. These can be particularly helpful in the assessment of comorbid sexual dysfunctions in the client and in her partner, case conceptualization, and treatment monitoring (for a comprehensive description of these measures and the best use of them, see Meana et al., 2008).

Medical/physical therapy evaluations. Finally, if the client has been referred for a medical or physical therapy evaluation, information from the client's treating physician or physical therapist with respect to results from laboratory tests (e.g., for hormone function, vascular integrity, and nerve function) and physical examinations (e.g., gynecological and pelvic floor assessment) will provide useful information for treatment.

Education

Although clients tend to be much more sexually savvy than they were 40 years ago when Masters and Johnson started treating sexual problems, ignorance, misinformation, and myths about sex continue to abound. Many clients have little understanding of both the physical and subjective aspects of female sexual arousal, and most know nothing about sexual pain. In addition, there are persistent beliefs that work to make both men and women feel inadequate sexually (e.g., that men should always be ready for sex, that women should reach orgasm through intercourse, that the couple should reach orgasm simultaneously, and that sex should always be spontaneous). It is not uncommon for clients to have idealized, media-propagated notions of ideal sex. Finally, many clients fail to grasp the ways in which physical and psychological factors interact. Not surprisingly, the general public continues to espouse the dichotomous view of sexuality that has been generally propagated, wherein problems are labeled either physical or psychological. Education is, thus, an important component of treating the woman with sexual difficulties, as well as her partner.

Despite the ubiquitous presence of sexual themes in contemporary media, misinformation and myths about sex abound

Education is the base from which to establish reasonable expectations and to target cognitive distortions that will continue to flare up throughout the core treatment phase. It is also the base from which to set realistic treatment goals. The client also needs to be educated about what her treatment options are. Clients are often anxious about the treatment of sexual problems (many people still believe that sex therapy involves the use of surrogates). Clearing up these misconceptions as early as possible is recommended. In addition, treatment options within the concurrent multidisciplinary model may be quite varied and run the gamut from communication skills to surgery. The client needs to know what these are before committing to treatment goals and strategies. Clinician-imparted knowledge can also be augmented with appropriate self-help resources that can be help facilitate the transfer of treatment gains to the home setting (van Lankveld, 2009). (See Section 6 for a list of self-help resources for women and their partners.)

Clearly, the concurrent multidisciplinary model also requires that the clinician educate him or herself about a variety of treatments that fall outside their area of applied competence. This is particularly true if they are going to work with other health care professionals as a team. Staying conversant with the female sexual dysfunction treatment outcome literature is essential.

Assessing Readiness for Change

The treatment for sexual difficulties can be quite challenging for clients. It is common to witness a pattern of avoidance in all of the sexual dysfunctions. Sex has become problematic, and the client has probably developed a complex series of strategies to get around it. It is also often a source of discord in the couple, and they may have become quite adept at sidestepping the issue. Therapy is likely to take them in the opposite direction. Both sex and couple issues will be confronted and engaged. At the beginning, that can be a strain, and different clients will have different levels of motivation for change. There may also be a discrepancy between the woman's motivation for change in her sexual life and that of her partner. Both are likely to have a major impact on treatment.

The transtheoretical model of Prochaska and Prochaska (1999) posits that clients vary in their motivation for change and that treatment is most likely to be effective if it is matched to the client's "change stage." The five stages of the model with a direct applicability to sex therapy are precontemplation, contemplation, preparation, action, and maintenance. In the *precontemplation* stage, the client has not yet entirely acknowledged that there is a problem. If one of the partners is in this stage, the therapy will likely have to proceed lightly with the aim being to help the client or her partner consider how their lives might improve with change. In the *contemplation* stage, the problem is acknowledged but the client is not sure she wants to change or if she is capable of it. For example, a woman with low desire may know it is problematic but be reticent to reengage sexually or lack faith that anything will work. In these cases it is important not to pressure the client. In the *preparation* stage, the treatment plan is likely to shift into a more active gear that builds up the client's self-efficacy. When clients commit to change, the *action* stage commences and behavioral activation is likely to be a major component of treatment. In the *maintenance* stage, a consolidation of therapy gains is undertaken and plans are made for the possible recurrence of problems.

A skillful assessment of the woman's and her partner's stages of change is essential to the construction of realistic treatment goals. Motivational interviewing techniques are specifically designed to assess motivation for change (Miller & Rollnick, 1991). Although some motivational deficits will only arise later in the therapy when the treatment intensifies, a good motivational interview early on will likely be very useful, especially when there are motivational discrepancies in a couple. Failing to take motivation for change into account can quickly lead to treatment impasses and the unhelpful labeling of the client as treatment resistant.

> Assessing a client's stage of readiness for treatment can provide helpful information for treatment planning

Goal Setting

For the most part, the setting of goals in the treatment of sexual problems is not particularly different from the setting of goals for any other type of therapy. They should be collaboratively generated, realistic, as well defined as possible, measurable, stated in positive terms, matching the client's stage of readiness for change, and meaningful. However, the ultimate goal of therapy for sexual problems is sexual and relationship satisfaction, rather than a specific desire level, arousal level, or frequency of orgasms.

There is a wide diversity in what we call sexual function and the only thing that really matters is whether the woman and her partner feel comfortable with

The ultimate goal of therapy for sexual problems is sexual and relationship satisfaction

their sexuality, derive pleasure from the stimulation and intimacy of sex, and are contented with the emotional components of their sex life. Even in the case of dyspareunia, the goal of completely eradicating pain is often not achievable. In such a case, enhancing arousal, diversifying the couple's sexual repertoire (to reduce single-minded focus on penetration), and helping them reconnect sexually are all likely to significantly improve satisfaction, despite the pain still being present. Clients may at first be very attached to performance goals. It can be helpful to point out that performance goals are often at the root of sexual difficulties, and even when they are not, they can certainly interfere with sexual function. Thus, making performance the goal of therapy is likely to have the paradoxical effect of worsening the situation. Making pleasure, sensuality, and emotional closeness the goals of therapy is more likely to result in performance improvements.

Distress Reduction

Distress is as much anathema to sexual function as are performance goals. Although some distress (personal or interpersonal) is necessary for the client to seek help or to move along the readiness-for-change continuum, once the treatment starts, distress needs to be directly targeted and reduced. An immediate reduction in distress is likely to occur at the very beginning of therapy, partly as a function of the client knowing that they are actively seeking help and getting treatment. The therapist needs to capitalize on this by instilling hope, normalizing, helping generate attainable goals, and mediating the perceived or real impact of the sexual problem on the couple's nonsexual relationship.

Studies of the pharmacological treatment of women's sexual dysfunctions have documented a significant placebo effect (Bradford & Meston, 2009). Although a number of mechanisms have been invoked to explain the placebo response, it is thought to be largely a product of positive expectancy effects. Distinguishing placebo effects from "active ingredient" effects is complicated in psychotherapy. Some have even argued that psychotherapy itself is largely a placebo (Justman, 2011). In any case, there seems little question that when clients think they are engaging in a treatment that is going to help them, a significant number of them show immediate improvement.

This common response can be heightened by specific actions on the therapist's part. In addition to explicitly communicating hope while remaining realistic, therapist investment in results might enhance this natural tendency toward improvement when treatment is underway. Distress reduction can also be helped along by normalizing the client's problem. Because sex is rarely discussed truthfully, many clients and their partners have no idea that there are many women and couples having similar experiences. Knowing this can help to put the problem in perspective, decatastrophize it, and reduce associated distress about being "abnormal." The goal-setting exercise can also enhance self-efficacy by identifying satisfaction rather than mechanistic performance as the ultimate aim. Some women may not be able to relate to a sex frequency or orgasm goal, but most can imagine satisfaction.

Treatment that zeroes in on sexual satisfaction rather than sexual performance is likely to be more successful

Finally, many women who present with sexual difficulties are particularly distressed about the impact of the sexual problem on their relationship with a valued other. Fears of being left or "cheated on" abound, and more often than not, these anxieties are not expressed to the partner. Identifying the problem as a couple's problem (rather than just her problem) and having the partner become active in the treatment can go a long way toward reducing this type of anxiety. Suddenly the sexual issue becomes a team effort rather than one isolating the woman in her privately experienced doubts about her partner's commitment. Of course, there are cases in which the partner's commitment is insufficient to weather the difficulty, but the open avowal of this, terrifying though it can seem, usually beats living in fear of it happening.

Stage 2: Cognitive Restructuring, Emotional Regulation, Stimulus Control and Behavioral Activation, Relationship Skills Building

Cognitive Restructuring
After addressing the client's knowledge about sexual function as well as their early stage distress, the core treatment stage is likely to involve a continuing effort to target maladaptive thoughts and to regulate emotions surrounding the sexual concern. Among the most useful cognitive strategies reported are sex script modification, cognitive restructuring, and techniques to enhance one's perception of desirability.

Sex script modification. Many maladaptive thoughts can be linked to sexual scripts. The client or couple comes in with an ideal of how sex should feel or how it should progress; an ideal they are not attaining. Sometimes both partners share the same script, and sometimes there are significant script discrepancies. Deviations from these scripts often result in distressing thoughts about the self and about the relationship. Frequent thoughts relating to the self have to do with themes of inadequacy, abnormality, illness, loss of control, and lack of attractiveness or desirability. Common distressing themes relating to the relationship include the partner's lack of attraction, his/her judgment, negative comparisons with previous partners, as well as fears of infidelity, abandonment, and lack of love. Relationship-related cognitive distortions can flourish in the case of sexual dysfunction because most couples do not often talk seriously about sex. This can be especially true when sex is problematic. The avoidance of the topic thus becomes fertile ground for the proliferation of beliefs about the partner's feelings that may have little basis in fact. Even if the sexual dysfunction does not originate in cognitive and emotional disturbances, there seems little doubt that negative cognitions and affect regarding the self or the relationship will exacerbate the problem.

Targeting maladaptive thoughts. Scripts can be elicited from clients quite directly by simply asking them to describe their ideal, acceptable, or unacceptable sexual scenarios. More specific cognitions can be identified and tracked with standard cognitive monitoring forms custom-tailored to sexual interactions. The client and partner can keep a sex diary wherein they identify thoughts and associated emotions in the context of any type of sexual activity (from the verbal suggestion to have sex, to kissing, to intercourse). As in any of other type of CBT, the clinician can then start the work of challenging distortions when and if they occur, have members of the couple challenge each other's distortions, and finally work with both of them to generate more factual and less catastrophic cognitions. Along with a number of other behavioral strategies, this process can instill a sense of self-efficacy in the management of the sexual difficulty so that, at the very least, the client and his/her partner no longer feel helpless.

Fantasy can be used to enhance arousal

Sexual imagery and fantasy. The use of sexual imagery and fantasy is another set of cognitive strategies commonly reported in the sex therapy literature. Just as helping people think adaptive thoughts reduces distress and catastrophization, helping people think sexy thoughts can enhance desire and arousal. Distraction away from sexual stimuli has consistently been linked to sexual dysfunction, and women with low desire report being distracted during sex. Rather than focusing on sexual stimuli, they find themselves thinking about their to-do list; this is clearly not an ideal cognitive condition for sexual enjoyment. Cognitively refocusing clients on sexual stimuli either before or during sex can have significant positive effects, regardless of the dysfunction. It is not uncommon, however, for clients to need permission to engage in sexual fantasy, as some women fear that fantasizing may be a form of infidelity, especially if the fantasy does not include their partner.

Encourage women to engage in self-care and other behaviors that make them feel sexy

Sexual self-concept. Sexual self-concept is another important cognitive schema that might require intervention. There is evidence that a woman's own sense of her sexual desirability may be significantly linked to sexual function and satisfaction (Andersen & Cyranowski, 1994). One study of married women with low desire found that a majority of them had ceased to consider themselves sexual beings. This was especially true of mothers with young children (Sims & Meana, 2010). If a woman has stopped considering herself attractive or sexually desirable, the impact on her desire and responsiveness is likely to be negative. Exploring a women's sexual self-concept, and targeting distortions therein, can be a fruitful avenue for the instatement of desire and arousal. Activation of behavioral strategies that make the woman feel better about herself or sexier is also recommended. Every woman will identify a different set of behaviors likely to affect her sexual self-concept. For some it may involve reengaging in physical exercise; for others it may be shopping for lacy lingerie; for yet others it may involve engaging in social situations that do not involve family duties. Women generally have a good idea about what makes them feel sexy and what does not.

Emotional Regulation

Although the targeting of maladaptive thoughts and schema is ultimately aimed at the reduction of distress, emotion may also need to be targeted directly. Strategies focused directly on emotion generally involve affective awareness, emotional regulation training, relaxation/mindfulness, and acceptance.

Affective awareness. Some couples will present with high levels of negative emotion about the sexual problem. Others, afraid of the potential threat of negative emotion to the relationship or to their partner's feelings, will suppress emotion. Neither scenario is helpful to the resolution or management of the sexual problem. A first order of business for both the clinician and the couple is thus to get a real sense of the emotional landscape within which the sexual dysfunction is operating. Before emotions are targeted, everyone has to know what they are. Developing affective awareness is as important to the treatment effort as cognitive awareness is.

Modulating emotions/anxiety reduction. Cases characterized by emotionally focused coping can result in anger, hostility, mood disturbances, and even sexual aversion. These strong emotions can make clients feel helpless and out of control, and they can work to entrench the sexual difficulty. Helping the client and her partner modulate emotional reactivity can reduce stress and help them progress through treatment. A large number of relaxation techniques (e.g., progressive muscle relaxation, deep breathing, and guided imagery) have long been used in clinical psychology to reduce anxiety and distress related to any number of conditions.

Although these can be useful adjuncts to therapy for sexual problems, emotional regulation is probably best served by adopting a different stance in regard to the imagined inevitability and reliability of emotions. Clients are often under the impression that emotions are uncontrollable and that they necessarily signal some truth that must be attended to. Disabusing clients of these beliefs can be effective in helping them gain control of destructive emotional states that serve to exacerbate the sexual problem. Over the course of therapy, the integration of the following precepts of emotional regulation can be helpful to the client who is a prisoner of maladaptive emotion-focused coping:
(1) Emotional reactions are often within your control.
(2) Feeling something does not make it true.
(3) It is not always useful to submit to and go with a feeling.
(4) You can choose to feel something different and more constructive.

These principles of emotional regulation can turn the experience of a less-than-perfect sexual interaction from a catastrophic event signaling personal inadequacy or relationship incompatibility, to a constructive, incremental step toward sexual fulfillment, some components of which were satisfying.

> **Reducing emotional reactivity is central to navigating the ups and downs of a sex life, as well as the ups and downs of treatment**

The most prominent emotion in both male and female sexual dysfunctions is anxiety. As per Barlow's model, anxiety competes with sexual stimuli, and when it wins, sexual difficulties ensue. The anxiety can be about performance (arousal or orgasm), or about disappointing a partner, or about sexual self-concept, or about perceived norms of sexual desire or behavior, or it can be about pain. Anxiety about sex comes in many shapes and sizes. All variants, however, tend to interfere with function, pleasure, and satisfaction. As such, identifying the sources of the anxiety and targeting associated cognitions is a central aspect of the treatment for sexual difficulties.

Acceptance. One aspect of emotional regulation that has been receiving increasing theoretical and empirical attention is the concept of acceptance, a practice rooted in Buddhism and Eastern philosophies. Represented in the general literature primarily by acceptance and commitment therapy (ACT), dialectical behavior therapy (DBT), and mindfulness-based cognitive therapy (MCT), acceptance relates primarily to the defusing of thoughts, emotions, memories, and experiences so that we neither struggle with them nor have them define who we are. Extrapolating to a sex therapy context, acceptance is useful both in the regulation of emotions but also in helping clients live with limitations that may not be within their control. Not all negative thoughts about

> **Accepting limitations is as important as embracing change where change is possible**

sexuality will be distortions. Not all clients will be able to achieve the sexual function they wish they had – either because of age or other physical and/or psychological limitations. Not all couples can have the desires of both partners met, sexual or nonsexual. Most will not. Acceptance of certain realities can be just as positively impactful as attempts to change what can indeed be modified.

Mindfulness. One acceptance-related therapy modality that shows promise for the treatment of sexual problems in women is mindfulness meditation. The practice of mindfulness consists of exercises designed to decrease distracting, negative, and anxiety-producing cognitions that prevent individuals from being fully engaged in the present moment. Brotto and colleagues (2008) have reported positive outcomes in a treatment protocol for women with desire and arousal problems. Their protocol added mindfulness to more traditional sex therapy components such as cognitive-behavioral exercises, psychoeducation, and communication skills training. In two separate studies, participant feedback indicated that mindfulness was perceived to be the most impactful component of treatment. There are a number of general resources that instruct on the practice of mindfulness meditation (see Section 6).

Stimulus Control and Behavioral Activation

Although the woman and her partner's thoughts and emotions are likely to be important contributors to the sexual experience, external factors can be as important as internal ones. The arousal of even the most well-adjusted and sex-positive woman will, for the most part, require competent sexual stimuli and contexts. However, in the case of sexual difficulties, it is common for the stimuli to be impaired or misperceived. Therapy then has to adopt a double focus both on the internal world of the client and on the external circumstances during which sex occurs or does not occur. Common stimulus control strategies used with all or most sexual dysfunctions are genital self-exploration, directed masturbation, sensate focus, and optimization of timing and context.

Genital self-exploration. Some women have little knowledge of, or comfort with, their genitalia. This proportion is likely to be higher among the population of women struggling with sexual problems. Unlike male genitalia, female genitalia are not exposed to the same extent and require some effort to explore. In addition, societal messages about female genitalia continue to be negatively framed, making many women uncomfortable with this part of their own bodies. Both the lack of knowledge and the queasiness can interfere with sexual enjoyment. If a woman does not know her own physiology, it can be difficult to communicate stimulation preferences to a partner. In addition, if she has a negative genital self-image, this is likely to interfere both cognitively and emotionally with the sexual experience. In a recent nationally representative sample of 3,800 US women ages 18–60, genital self-image was significantly related to sexual function and genital health care behaviors (Herbenick et al., 2011).

Genital self-exploration exercises can be helpful in targeting lack of knowledge about genitalia, as well as building comfort and appreciation for this part of the woman's own body. Generally, these consist of directing the woman to examine herself with a mirror and become acquainted with the location, tissue texture, and sensitivity of different parts of her genitals. Although women are subjected to much genital observation via a lifetime of gynecological examinations, a special effort is required for women to actually see themselves. Not all clients will require this intervention, but it can be helpful in women dealing with negative attitudes about sex or with arousal and orgasm difficulties.

Directed masturbation. Related to genital exploration is the technique of directed masturbation. Most often applied to cases of lifelong anorgasmia, it can also be useful in cases of low desire and arousal. It involves guiding the woman to self-educate in possible ways to achieve orgasm. Through exploratory self-stimulation, the woman can ascertain what types of stimulation she enjoys. Along with genital self-exploration, directed masturbation helps women discover what is and is not arousing for them. Women are asked to attend to bodily sensations (not just genital ones), to monitor and adjust maladaptive thoughts that might accompany masturbation or any sexual stimulation, and to experiment with sexual fantasies. By removing the relational component of sex, the woman has the opportunity to truly focus on sensations. She does not have to worry about what her partner is thinking, about how long she is taking to achieve orgasm, and/or about having to pleasure him or her. What she learns from directed masturbation can serve to improve solitary sex, but the aim is usually to transfer the knowledge and skills to partnered sexual activity.

Sensate focus. While genital self-exploration and directed masturbation are techniques primarily designed to improve the competence of sexual stimulation, sensate focus relates more directly to the concept of stimulus control. Regardless of the presenting sexual complaint, it is often the case that by the time couples seek help, their sexual interactions are malfunctioning on many levels. In these cases, it may be helpful to press the proverbial reset button and start a type of sexual retraining that de-emphasizes performance and focuses on sensuality.

> Sensate focus takes the couple back to the pleasure and sensuality of sex and away from anxiety-producing performance demands

Introduced by Masters and Johnson (1970) and refined by Kaplan (1974), sensate focus attempts to do just that. It takes the couple back to the pleasures of sensual touch and then sequentially through a series of structured and custom-tailored homework exercises that gradually move across the sexual intensity continuum. Sexual intercourse or stimulation aimed at producing orgasm (in the self or in the partner) is usually discouraged or banned at the start of sensate focus. On one hand, this retraining serves to refocus the couple on the central aim of sexuality – giving and receiving pleasure. On the other hand, sensate focus also works as a form of systematic desensitization. The anxiety attached to the sexual difficulty is immediately defused by an explicit turning away from performance demands, which are generally at the heart of the anxiety. The couple then progresses through the steps in the custom-tailored hierarchy at whatever pace is comfortable for them emotionally. Generally speaking, there are three phases in sensate focus: nongenital pleasuring, genital pleasuring, and intercourse or other orgasm producing sexual activity (see Table 6 for a brief description in the case of intercourse).

A number of authors have described the individual steps in a sensate focus hierarchy (Hawton, 1985; Kaplan, 1974; Masters & Johnson, 1970), but flexibility is the operative word. As in the treatment of any anxiety concern, the

Table 6
Sensate Focus Procedures

Stage	Exercises	Instructions to clients	In-session explanation and review
Nongenital pleasuring	Clothed, semiclothed, or naked caressing or other nongenital contact (holding hands, French kissing, etc.)	1. Focus on pleasure alone 2. Do not make orgasm a goal 3. Attend to sensation of being touched and of touching	1. Explain clearly the purpose of sensate focus 2. Do not ask client about whether orgasm happened during exercise 3. Focus on how they felt 4. Check on barriers to pleasure 5. Identify pleasure facilitators
Genital pleasuring	Extension of caressing to genital areas and breasts	1–3 4. Keep the caressing gentle	2–5 6. If orgasm is reported, do not focus on it as outcome success
Intercourse	Gradual reintroduction of activity	1–3 5. Containment without thrusting[a] 6. Woman controls depth & pace 7. Thrusting is reintroduced gradually 8. Experimentation with positions	2–6

Note. [a]*Containment* refers to penetration without partner thrusting. The woman controls depth of the penetration, and she is the one who moves to determine the depth and pace of the penetration.

hierarchy needs to be designed in collaboration with the client. The goals of each stage also need to be explicit and clearly understood. Failure to heed the client's anxiety by creating too accelerated a pace, and/or failure to explain the purpose of the exercises can result in noncompliance, an increase in anxiety, and renewed avoidance. If the client or her partner is overwhelmed by one of the steps, then it is wise to step back and perhaps introduce another level of gradation to the hierarchy. Sensate focus exercises often surprise both clients and clinicians, as they can be quite diagnostic in revealing anxieties and fears that had not been identified.

Weeks and Gambescia (2009) suggest that the nine functions of sensate focus are to:

(1) help each partner become more aware of her or his own sensations;
(2) focus on one's own needs for pleasure and worry less about the problem or the partner;
(3) communicate sensual and sexual needs, wishes, and desires;
(4) increase awareness of the partner's sensual and sexual needs;
(5) expand the repertoire of intimate, sensual behaviors;
(6) learn to appreciate foreplay as a goal start rather than a means to an end;
(7) create positive relational experiences;
(8) build sexual desire;
(9) enhance the level of love, caring, commitment, intimacy, cooperation, and sexual interest in the relationship.

This is a tall order indeed and unlikely to be achieved by sensate focus alone. However, keeping these ideal functions in mind can be helpful in the collaborative design of the sensate focus exercises.

Optimizing timing and context. One final stimulus control feature applicable to the treatment of any couple with sexual problems relates to the optimization of timing and context. Although good timing and favorable conditions enhance the sexual experience of all couples, they are particularly important to women and couples experiencing sexual problems. The literature seems fairly clear in its finding that women generally have more sexual arousal contingencies than do men. Factors such as mood, stress, fatigue, and general context appear to have more of an impact on women's desire and arousal than on that of men. Many men may not understand this greater arousal contingency in women, leading to hurtful misinterpretations of refused advances. In addition, couples with sexual problems are probably more likely to make timing and context errors, as frustration has set in, and sexual demands can issue forth thoughtlessly or even in anger.

Examining the context in which sex is either proposed or happens may be very helpful to the treatment effort. A common report by working couples with or without children is that by the time they get to bed, they are too tired to have sex. Sex becomes secondary and is not prioritized, despite its importance to the relationship. Another common problem is sexual advances made when either member of the couple is stressed or in a hurry (Sims & Meana, 2010). Helping the couple understand each other's arousal contingencies, respect them, and then agree to have sex when reasonable conditions are met will nurture desire, arousal, and orgasmic capacity. This may be particularly important for women, whose arousal appears to be more context-dependent. On the other hand, if arousal contingencies are numerous and difficult to achieve, it may signal desire and arousal problems.

One of the reasons that couples fall into the difficulty of initiating or having sex at the wrong times is that, over time, they tend to relegate sex to a secondary status, well behind jobs, parenting, and other important life responsibilities. Most couples report that this happened incrementally and often imperceptibly. The result is that no time is reserved for sex. Rather, sex is awkwardly wedged in between other activities. This type of situation generally requires intervention.

Good sex requires
both time and
attention

Making time for sex is important for all couples, but particularly for couples struggling with sexual difficulties. Sex needs attention, and it needs to be prioritized. How couples decide to do that, with clinician guidance, will vary. Scheduling time for sex does go up against the powerful spontaneity script to which many clients are attached. On the other hand, most will agree that waiting for spontaneity is not working out for them. Some clients will want to schedule a preordained time for sex, while others will commit to making the time without a rigid schedule. Either way, the aim is to make clients aware that they have to start prioritizing sex sufficiently to make it happen under positive circumstances. Waiting for "spontaneous combustion" or wedging sex in between two stressors can only further complicate existing difficulties.

Expanding the sexual repertoire. Many long-term couples complain of mechanistic sex consisting of predefined steps in a rigid sexual script. Typically, nonpenetrative activities are dismissively considered foreplay, and the main event is defined as sexual intercourse, for heterosexual couples, or another orgasm-aimed finale, for same-sex couples. These routines can become boring over time, even if they end up providing stimulation adequate for orgasm. Encouraging clients to mix up scripts and try new forms of stimulation or intercourse positions can reinvigorate tired sex that even sexually functional couples have lost enthusiasm for. With the clinician's help and with a focus on preferences rather than dislikes, couples can educate each other about things they would like to try, as well as give each other permission to experiment. The consensual broadening of sexual scripts and collaborative exploration of sexual activities outside of the regular routine can render sex more exciting. This in turn can have a salutatory effect on desire, arousal, and orgasm. In the case of women with dyspareunia, removing the focus from penetrative sex can open up stimulating sexual interactions that are not overshadowed by the necessary anticipation of penetration-related pain.

Using erotica and sexual aids. The use of erotica in the form of books or videos, as well as vibrators or other sexual aids, can also enhance arousal for some women and couples. However, this is an intervention that needs to be approached gingerly as some individuals have strong moral or cultural concerns about using such materials. Erotica can be used by the individual woman in an attempt to enhance arousal or by the couple together in anticipation of, or during, sex. There are some points of potential sensitivity though. First, there is a wide variation in erotica and some is surely to be distasteful, especially to women. Viewing erotica can also be experienced by both partners as a form of infidelity, wherein the arousal is attributed to an outside image instead of the partner. There are also concerns about a growing dependence on this type of stimulation and its impact on real sexual interactions. The clinician can start by simply asking the couple to determine whether or not they would be open to erotica as an adjunct to therapy. If couples are willing to experiment, then there is a wealth of materials for the clients to research in bookstores, sex stores, video distributors, and on the Internet.

In a recent nationally representative study of 3,800 American women ages 18–60, 52.5% reported using vibrators, and vibrator use was positively associated with all aspects of sexual function as well as with health-promoting behaviors (Herbenick et al., 2009). Female clients who have never used a vibrator may benefit from exploring its integration into both solitary and partnered sex. Again, there may be some sensitivities associated with the suggestion. Some women may feel uncomfortable for any variety of cultural issues, and there may be concerns about dependence on the vibrator for arousal. Partners may also feel threatened by the arousal not emanating directly from their stimulation. Consequently, clinicians will first want to discuss attitudes about vibrator use before making it a part of the intervention.

Lifestyle modification. There are also general lifestyle factors than can interfere with sexual function. Studies repeatedly show that general health is related to sexual function. A frank and general discussion with clients about lifestyle factors can engender changes that help the client well beyond their sexual dysfunction. Among these factors are stress, exercise, smoking, and alcohol or other substance use. Stress is a particularly endemic problem as it bridges both physical and psychological well-being in ways that are evident to clients. Most men and women will agree that stress is anathema to engaged and positive sexual interactions. General lifestyle factors are often difficult to change, and it is unlikely that much of the therapy for the sexual problem will be spent directly on these. However, opening the discussion and educating the client about the possible sexual ramifications of these aspects of their lives can result in the client undertaking other measures to address them (e.g., joining a gym, taking up yoga, dieting, and/or taking less work home).

> **Healthy lifestyle changes can lead to better sexual function**

Relationship Skills Building
Regardless of the sexual dysfunction the woman may be encountering, relationship factors are likely to be an important component of the treatment effort. The nature of the association between the sexual difficulty and nonsexual aspects of the relationship (if one exists) is sometimes immediately obvious, but it often reveals itself more gradually as treatment progresses. The therapist will thus have to adjust to address emerging relational issues. It is important, however, to keep in mind that not all couples with sexual problems have relational maladjustment related to the problem. There are essentially (1) happy couples in which one or both have a sexual dysfunction, (2) partners who have significant problems relating to each other on levels that are unrelated to their sexual interaction, and (3) partners whose levels of attraction to each other, resentment, or myriad other relational conflicts are seriously interfering with sex. In all cases, relationship skills building will be necessary to the extent that treatment for sexual problems often requires couples to reengage in ways that are either new or long forgotten.

Relationship-targeted interventions range from macroexplorations of relational dynamics to more microbehavioral directives for communication about sexual likes and dislikes. It is in the relationship component of treatment that we witness the broadest theoretical integration, as interventions draw from psychodynamic principles and attachment theory, as well as from strict behaviorism. Couples whose relationship is in distress over and above the sexual difficulty are more likely to require in-depth work, while well-adjusted couples will be helped by specific techniques. This section starts with the broader interventions aimed at the more complex couple dynamics and moves to simpler

> **Sexual problems are not always rooted in maladjusted relationships; happy couples can also experience difficulty**

ones that can be helpful for all couples. The reason for the order lies in an important therapeutic reality. Couples whose relationship has deteriorated to the point where trust and respect are very low will be unlikely to tolerate more specific behavioral techniques to improve their sex life.

Individuation/differentiation. Building on principles from object relations and attachment theories, Schnarch (2003) makes a compelling case for the importance of differentiation to positive sexual interactions. In this iteration, the core conflict that paralyzes many couples lies in narcissistic fragility or insecurity. The couple who presents with conflict or as having lost a connection to each other is likely enmeshed rather than distant. One partner's well-being is overly dependent on the other partner's responses. Neither is sufficiently securely attached to the other to be able to truly listen and empathize with their partner's experiences, without ruminating about how these negatively reflect on them.

Intimacy may be hampered by inability to self-soothe and unrealistic reliance on each other for personal well-being

Through this solitary lens of self-defense, a partner's sexual dysfunction is a threat to self; for example, the partner of the woman with low desire might think her low desire reflects her lack of attraction for him/her (which may or may not be true), engendering anger, resentment, or disengagement. The woman with low desire, in turn, might expect that its resolution lies in his/her hands (the other person needs to do more housework, romance me more, etc. – which may in part be true, or not at all). Partner problems are overrelated to the self (personalized), and the resolution of self problems are unreasonably expected to emanate from the other. Members of such couples are unrealistically charged with each other's well-being. Under such conditions, intimacy is impossible.

In the couple characterized by such a dynamic, the treatment of sexual difficulties will be facilitated by an awareness of this dynamic, the challenging of narcissistic interpretations of sexual interactions, the generation of mutual responsibility for dynamics, and the promotion of self-soothing and self-intervention to incrementally replace the damaging reliance on the partner for well-being. Such couples often present with long lists of complaints about the other and can easily generate equally long lists of required improvements from the other. A key intervention here is to have them generate such lists for themselves rather than for their partners: What have they done less than well? What improvements can they make and are willing to commit to? Making each member of the couple responsible for and actively engaged in their self-improvement is likely to yield better results than the mutual exchange of desired change in the other.

Shifting each individual's focus from partner blame to self-improvement is likely to result in better outcomes

Conflict resolution. The refocusing of responsibility on the self rather than on the other can have a positive effect on conflict resolution, as it defuses blame. However, occasional conflict is a natural component of most relationships. Learning how to navigate it successfully can significantly reduce the amount of time a couple wastes on negative interactions and can increase the probability of both positive interactions and sexual ones. Gottman (1999) identified four ways of relating that engender conflict: criticism, defensiveness, contempt, and stonewalling. The most empirically validated maladaptive pattern of relating, commonly witnessed in the context of sexual difficulties (especially in cases of HSDD), is the demand–withdrawal pattern (Heavey, Christensen, &

Malamuth, 1995). In this pattern of relating, one partner insists on having his or her "needs" met, while the other reacts to this insistence by withdrawing. The more the latter withdraws, the more the former demands, and the more the former demands, the more the latter withdraws.

Women with low desire often describe situations in which partners make frequent demands for sex, which make them increasingly avoidant, which in turn makes the appeals more desperate and the avoidance more pronounced. As obvious as this pattern can be to a third party, couples are often unaware that they are stuck in a cycle of behavior that gets both of them more of exactly what they do not want. Making couples aware of their patterns regarding sexual and other conflict can have an immediate disabling effect on the maladaptive pattern. Suddenly they see it happening, when before, they were unaware.

Breaking circular patterns of sexual avoidance and sexual demands is crucial to treatment

Testing out a different pattern and realizing that they get more of what they want can be a powerful intervention. If the partner of the woman with low desire notices that when he or she demands less, the woman either initiates more often or is more responsive when they make an advance, then the partner is likely to continue this less demanding strategy. Likewise if the woman notices that less avoidance results in fewer demands, she might avoid less. That is, at least, the principle. There will be cases in which the decrease in demands will be met with relief and no less avoidance. In any case, helping clients learn how to resolve conflicts more effectively and reduce the recovery time from the inevitable resurgence of conflict can have a positive effect on their sexual lives.

Increasing nonsexual affection. Positive sexual experiences are facilitated by positive nonsexual experiences. One can even conceptualize sex as the culmination of positive nonsexual experiences with a sexual partner. Women certainly endorse that their desire for sex increases when sex is not the one solitary act of intimacy between them and their partners. Couples with sexual difficulties have often stopped touching each other or expressing nonsexual affection.

There can be many reasons for this. Men and women appear to differ in their nonsexual intimacy needs and in their interpretation of sexual cues. This gender difference, left unexplored and discussed, can result in misunderstandings and dissatisfaction. Women may come to fear that any type of physical affection risks being misinterpreted as a sexual advance. If the woman is avoiding sex, as many women with sexual difficulties do, she will then be reticent to physically demonstrate affection, for fear that her partner will misread the touch, kiss, or hug. She will also be likely to reject, or tense up at, demonstrations of affection from her partner. However, this is a vicious cycle, as it engenders a nonphysical interaction pattern that women themselves report as not being conducive to sexual desire.

Increasing nonsexual physical affection can be an effective intervention. However, it is paradoxical in nature. On the one hand, the clinician will want to make a clear distinction between physical affection and sexual advances so that physical affection feels safe. On the other hand, one of the aims of this increase in physical affection (other than the sheer pleasure and emotional intimacy) is to set up conditions over time that will ultimately facilitate positive sexual interactions. Some couples have to relearn how to be nonsexually affectionate, but this is one of the easier and most welcomed interventions.

Romantic activation. Related to the increase in nonsexual affection is the activation or reactivation of romance in the relationship. Romantic interactions are here generally defined as interactions communicating sexual desire for a whole person rather than desire simply for sex or for contact with a body part. They are generally personal, thoughtful, and artful rather than merely sexually explicit. Research has consistently found that women report a strong preference for sexual interactions that incorporate romantic elements, signaling that the sexual desire is person-specific (Graham et al., 2004; Sims & Meana, 2010). Although men may be more focused on sexual explicitness than romantic scenarios, they also appear to enjoy and value that type of attention (Janssen et al., 2008).

Unfortunately, romance has a tendency to decline in long-term relationships, and this is likely to negatively impact the sexual satisfaction of both men and women, although the effect may be particularly salient for the latter. Couples are often buried under responsibilities, and familiarity has a tendency to dampen expressions of desire and appreciation of the partner. Before long, a couple whose courtship and early years together were romantic and sexy has turned into little more than roommates. Not uncommonly, sex has also become mechanistic and sexual advances crude and unimaginative.

The good news is that both men and women generally welcome interventions that increase the level of romance in the relationship. This type of intervention has to be collaboratively designed with clients, as there is great variation in what individuals find sexy and romantic. It is also likely that the couple will have to educate each other about what they would like to see happen. The clinician can make suggestions for ways to promote romanticism if the couple is stumped (e.g., loving phone or text messages, cards, dates, more prolonged and sensitive foreplay, etc.), but these are likely to be more effective if they are generated by the clients. Client generation of ideas will also help to defuse the potential for these new or revisited strategies to feel staged and inauthentic.

Enhancing communications skills. When you ask couples how often they talk seriously about sex, it is common to hear "rarely" or "never", even from couples who have been together for many years. Aside from the general societal discomfort with sexuality, sex is an interpersonally sensitive topic. It involves a high level of vulnerability and exposure (so to speak), which likely makes individuals particularly sensitive to offense or rejection. When interviewed without their partners, women will often describe enduring sexual stimulation they dislike, for fear of hurting their partner's feelings. Furthermore, research indicates that between one half and two thirds of women have faked orgasm, with a prominent reason being an attempt to spare the partner's feelings (Muehlenhard & Shippee, 2010). Understandable and laudable though the consideration of the partner's sensitivities is, no one is ultimately served by silence about sexual preferences and dislikes.

The fear of hurting a partner's feelings can lead to years of enduring ineffective sexual stimulation

Treating the sexually dysfunctional couple often requires helping them communicate about sex honestly, respectfully, and with a focus on correction rather than complaint. Following the spirit of depersonalizing sexual issues, couples can be instructed in the positive communication of sexual preferences. As aforementioned, this is an integral component of the sensate focus exercises. Although clients should be consulted on ways in which they would prefer this type of communication to occur, there are at least three interventions that can be suggested:

(1) *Mutual corrective feedback*: After a sexual episode, each individual can identify two things the partner did that were very arousing and two things that were less than satisfying. It is important that both members of the couple be required to engage in the exercise so as to remove the feared elements of blame and hurt. The feedback can then be acted on in the next sexual encounter so as to improve the experience.

(2) *Body shifts*: Talking is not the only way to communicate sexual preferences. The body is an effective communicator if the partner is attending. A minor shift or repositioning can be the adjustment needed to enhance pleasure or to communicate that a particular type of stimulation is not having the desired effect.

(3) *Hand-guiding*: Gently taking the partner's hand to model the stimulation desired can also be an effective nonverbal way of communicating the desired type and location of stimulation. This act can be performed as part of the lovemaking, without interruption.

Stage 3: Consolidation of Gains and Relapse Prevention
Psychological treatment of sexual difficulties can be an intense experience for couples. After months or years of avoiding discussion and direct action regarding sexual difficulties, they are thrown into a hothouse environment in which the taboo topic is focused on and addressed pointedly. Deep conversations are had and activities are planned as they never have been before. Change occurs and the couple can feel that they have conquered the problem. However, the gains made in therapy can fade over time as the spotlight on sexual interactions is removed and the usual pressures and predispositions start to seep back in. Changed circumstances and new stressors can also work to effect a backtracking into old patterns. None of this is unusual. As a matter of fact, it is to be expected. Consequently, it is helpful, prior to therapy termination, to review some of the dynamics that may have precipitated or maintained the sexual dilemma and to plan for potential relapses.

Below are some strategies to help prevent relapse that McCarthy (1993) and others have recommended:

(1) Review developmental origins of the problem, if these are identifiable.
(2) Instruct clients in the early identification of conditions that triggered or contributed to the problem so that they can address them before things get out of control or feel overwhelming.
(3) Encourage clients to devote the amount time they had spent in therapy on a weekly basis to touch base with each other on the status and quality of their connection (relational and/or sexual).
(4) Encourage the regular scheduling and establishment of enjoyable time together, alone.
(5) Encourage the continuation of sexual play that does not necessarily have orgasm as its goal.

(6) Plan follow-up therapy sessions for at least a year.
(7) Encourage clients to request booster sessions if they feel the need for a brief tune-up.

4.1.3   Dysfunction-Specific Assessment and Treatment Components

The previous section consisted of a generic template for the treatment of women/couples with sexual difficulties. Template components explicated basic interventions that can be generalized and applied across sexual dysfunctions. A number of those components have not been strictly empirically validated, either in combination or individually. Nonetheless, they constitute the nonspecific foundation of sexual dysfunction treatment endorsed by experienced sex therapists and currently practiced to varying degrees by a majority of practitioners.

In the following section, the empirically validated research for the specific assessment and treatment of each of the female sexual dysfunctions will be presented. The aim is for the reader to add or incorporate the dysfunction-specific assessment tools and interventions into the general template, depending on the presenting problem and its context. Although Masters and Johnson advocated the use of two therapists (the double-couple format wherein a therapist couple treated a patient couple), this mode of delivery has fallen out of favor. Psychological treatment delivery in the empirical research most commonly consists of an individual therapist working with a couple, or group therapy in which there is one therapist and a group of women or couples. The length of therapy varies across studies but averages somewhere between 8 and 12 weekly sessions. As in any other type of therapy, more complex cases may require longer treatment duration.

Hypoactive Sexual Desire Disorder

Assessment
Hypoactive sexual desire disorder (HSDD) can be difficult to diagnose as it is not anchored in the absence or disturbance of an expected discrete event (lubrication/orgasm) or in the presence of an unexpected one (pain during intercourse). Although most clinicians rely primarily on the clinical interview for the assessment of desire problems, self-administered measures can be a useful adjunct, and they can help monitor treatment progress. Table 7 provides a list of empirically validated self-report measures specifically targeting sexual desire. In addition, all global sexual function measures have desire scales (see Table 5).

In the absence of psychological, relational, situational, medication-related, or disease-related factors (see Table 4) that could reasonably account for decreases in sexual desire, it might be necessary to have the client assessed for hormone levels. Sexual desire in women appears to be more closely linked to testosterone than to estrogen, but it is important to keep in mind that no consistent correlations have been found between androgen levels and measures of desire and arousal (Davis et al., 2005).

Table 7
Self-Report Measures for the Assessment of Sexual Desire

Measure	Reference
For Use With Women and Men	
Sexual Desire Inventory (SDI)	Spector et al. (1996)
Hurlbert Index of Sexual Desire (HISD)	Apt & Hurlbert (1992)
For Use With Women	
Decreased Sexual Desire Screener (DSDS) *(assesses acquired HSDD)*	Clayton et al. (2009)
Sexual Interest and Desire Inventory – Female (SIDI-F)	Clayton et al. (2006); Sills et al. (2005)
Women's Sexual Interest Diagnostic Interview – Short Form (WSID-SF) *(to date validated for postmenopausal women only)*	Derogatis et al. (2010)
Menopausal Sexual Interest Questionnaire (MSIQ)	Rosen et al. (2004)
Profile of Female Sexual Function (PFSF) *(for naturally and surgically menopausal women)*	Derogatis et al. (2004)

Note. HSDD = Hypoactive Sexual Desire Disorder.

Psychological Treatment

Sexual desire problems are often invoked as the most difficult to treat of all of the sexual dysfunctions (except perhaps sexual pain). Research has certainly lagged behind the increasing demand for treatment. In their review of the literature since 2003, an expert committee recently gave the HSDD treatment outcome research effort a grade of C (Brotto, Bitzer, Laan, Leiblum, & Luria, 2010). Stretching back to 1991, there have only been a handful of HSDD outcome studies, broadly defined. Trudel and colleagues (2001) have been the only group to conduct a RCT with a follow-up of 1 year. These few published studies report success rates ranging from half to three quarters of women who completed treatment, although outcome measures varied widely and cross-study comparisons are close to impossible.

> Therapists can increase the reinforcing value of sex and improve the context in which sex takes place

The two major principles guiding the treatment of sexual desire have been (1) to increase the reinforcing value of sexual activity (e.g., increase arousal, orgasm, pleasure, physical, and emotional satisfaction), and (2) to improve the quality of nonsexual situations so as to facilitate the occurrence of sexual ones. All treatment components used in the empirical literature can be found in the generic treatment template provided in this text. The most common ones are sensate focus, sexual skills training, and communication skills training. In their group CBT, Trudel et al. (2001) also added analysis of immediate and long-term causal factors for the low desire, the provision of sexual information, emotional communication skills training, mutual reinforcements, cognitive restructuring, and fantasy training. Based on the principle that more consistent orgasms would lead to more desire, Hurlbert (1993) investigated orgasm consistency training as a treatment for HSDD and reported success. Orgasm consistency training consists of directed masturbation, the suggestion that the woman reach orgasm before her partner and before intercourse, and the coital alignment technique (finding positions in which the penis provides direct clitoral stimulation during intercourse).

The most recent treatment component empirically tested for the treatment of low sexual desire in women has been mindfulness-based CBT (Brotto et al., 2008). There is also some empirical support for the positive impact of marital therapy on sexual desire in women (MacPhee, Johnson, & van der Veer, 1995).

As the research indicates, low sexual desire is perhaps the most expansive of the female sexual dysfunctions in terms of its potential psychological causes and related complications (from comorbid sexual dysfunctions to relationship problems). Consequently, treatment for HSDD has also tended to include the largest number of psychological treatment components. Virtually all of the generic template treatment components covered in this text should at least be considered as part of a treatment plan. A specific combination and sequence of treatment components can then be tailored to the needs and circumstances of any one client.

Hormone Treatment

There is accumulating evidence that testosterone increases sexual desire in naturally and surgically menopausal women

The outcome research on the hormonal treatment of low desire has been funded to a greater extent than has psychological treatment and is consequently more voluminous. Hormone therapy (estrogen alone or estrogen-progestin) has been shown to reduce menopause–related sexual symptoms (e.g., lubrication deficits and dyspareunia), but its impact on sexual desire, arousal, and orgasmic response independent of its role in relieving menopausal symptoms is not supported by the majority of the evidence (Wierman et al., 2010). There is accumulating evidence that the addition of testosterone, however, does increase sexual desire in naturally and surgically menopausal women. In postmenopausal women with HSDD, transdermally delivered testosterone in conjunction with estrogen therapy, as well as without estrogen therapy, appears to produce positive sexual function changes, including increases in sexual desire. The effect of testosterone on premenopausal women is largely untested. One small study with premenopausal women with HSDD found improvements in sexual function and well-being (Goldstat et al, 2003). However, in premenopausal women, the administration of testosterone is likely to produce supraphysiological levels which are cause for concern (Wierman et al., 2010).

Testosterone has a greater effect on desire than does estrogen, but all women should be familiar with the risks involved

Despite its lack of official approval for the treatment of HSDD, many women seek testosterone therapy for distressing low desire, and many physicians suggest it or are willing to comply with these requests, at least on a short-term basis. Interested clients should be encouraged to have an in-depth discussion with their physicians about the possible risks of off-label testosterone treatment, dosing, delivery (e.g., oral versus transdermal), and duration. The risks are not yet well understood, but androgenic side effects such as hirsutism, acne, alopecia, insulin resistance, cardiovascular disease, metabolic syndrome, and breast cancer need to be considered and weighed against possible benefits. Women treated with testosterone should be monitored with annual breast and pelvic examinations, annual mammography, as well as lipid and metabolic profiles. Abnormal bleeding should also be evaluated.

Nonhormonal Medications

The central nervous system has been the main target of nonhormonal treatments for HSDD in women. Flibanserin, a failed antidepressant medication that acts as an agonist and as an antagonist to different serotonin receptors, appears to have a modest effect on sexual desire in women (Brotto et al., 2010). Anticipated by some as the female Viagra, the drug has not been approved for this use. Although flibanserin may be reconsidered in the future, published, peer-reviewed RCTs are needed, as are full evaluations of its safety. In women experiencing low desire induced by the use of SSRIs, the addition of bupropion (which blocks norepinephrine and dopamine reuptake) has been found to improve self-reported feelings of sexual desire (Clayton et al., 2004). The literature also contains some reports regarding the superiority of certain antidepressants in terms of reduced sexual side effects. These medications include mirtazapine, nefazodone, and reboxetine.

Sexual Aversion Disorder

Assessment

It is not unusual for sexual aversion disorder (SAD) to first present as HSDD. However, the aversion usually rises to the surface once exposure to sexual situations is introduced. Sensate focus, in addition to being a central treatment component for all of the sexual dysfunctions, also serves important assessment functions. Psychological and relational issues that were either not accessed or disclosed at intake often make their appearance during sensate focus exercises. This is particularly true for SAD, in which it can happen quite dramatically.

In terms of self-report measures, clients with SAD will score low on the desire-specific domains of the global sexual function measures or in the desire-specific measures, but it is unlikely that these will detect the severity of the problem. There is only one self-administered measure directly designed to assess sexual fear and avoidance: the Sexual Aversion Scale (SAS; Katz et al., 1989). This 30-item questionnaire assesses fears and phobic avoidance of sexual contact theorized to be associated with sexual trauma, guilt, social inhibitions, and fear of sexually transmitted diseases (STDs). Used primarily for research purposes, administration of the SAS might reduce delays in the discovery that what presented as low desire is actually something more intense. It could also prove useful in case conceptualization, as it can identify the source of the aversion.

Finally, because of the major role that anxiety plays in SAD, it is wise to assess for the presence of other types of anxiety disorder (especially panic disorder). The anxiety may be limited to sex, but SAD may be only one of a number of ways in which anxiety has taken hold of a woman's life.

Psychological Treatment

Unfortunately, there are no published treatment outcome studies for SAD and only a couple of brief case reports. Treatment recommendations thus emanate entirely from clinical experience and naturally draw heavily on the treatment principles for anxiety, panic, and simple phobias.

As phobic anxiety is at the center of SAD, it is recommended that treatment be focused on the reduction of this anxiety in an integrated fashion (Gold & Gold, 1993). From a cognitive standpoint, this starts with identification of the catastrophic thoughts that trigger the panic, followed by cognitive restructuring and possibly reinterpretation of somatic sensations. The cognitive restructuring is likely to be more complex in SAD cases involving sexual traumatization. Sexual trauma may never have been fully acknowledged or processed, and CBT interventions may have to pause, as needed, to deal with emotions surfacing with these realizations. Special attention may need to be devoted to issues of guilt, grief, and anger.

Be mindful of the possibility of relaxation-induced anxiety in the client with SAD

Stimulus control (behavioral) techniques are likely to be as central to the treatment of SAD as they are to other panic-related disorders. Sensate focus acts as the type of systematic desensitization recommended for panic, although the hierarchy of exercises is likely to require very fine gradation. In some cases, it might be indicated to have separate sets of hierarchies – one dealing with the woman's comfort in exploring her own body and another focused on partner relations (Finch, 2001). Relaxation techniques may have to be selected judiciously, as internally focused ones have been found to induce anxiety (relaxation-induced anxiety) in clients with certain panic disorders. Mindfulness techniques may be helpful, although this has yet to be tested empirically. Finally, if the client is partnered, relationship dynamics need to be assessed and addressed. The partner may unwittingly be playing a major role in the maintenance of the problem, and he or she will undoubtedly play a very significant one in the treatment.

Medications

Depending on the severity of the problem and the generalization of the anxiety, SSRIs may be indicated in the treatment of SAD. If the client experiences incapacitating symptoms of panic at even the lowest stages of genital self-exploration or sexual activity hierarchies, the prescription of an SSRI may be the anxiety reduction step needed to move forward with psychological treatment. Likewise, if the SAD is just one manifestation of widespread anxiety, an SSRI can be helpful on multiple levels. Of course, there is still the conundrum of SSRIs having a dampening effect on sexual desire. However, in the case of SAD, the first step is getting the client to *tolerate* sexual interactions. Once this has occurred, the next goal would be the instatement of sexual desire and pleasure. The treatment approach would then be as described above for HSDD, in addition to experimentation with pharmacological agents that have fewer sexual side effects.

Female Sexual Arousal Disorder

Assessment

Female sexual arousal disorder (FSAD) rarely presents in the absence of HSDD. Exceptions include menopausal women experiencing physiological changes affecting lubrication and discomfort with penetration, or women with a disease state or medication regimen that has similar effects on genital tissue and functionality.

There is no single self-administered questionnaire devoted exclusively to FSAD. However, most general sexual function measures and some sexual desire–specific measures include questions about arousal and lubrication (see Tables 5 and 7). The Sexual Function Questionnaire (SFQ) has the largest number of questions about arousal (eight questions), and it goes beyond the

DSM criteria for FSAD by attempting to distinguish between genital and sub-jective arousal. Physical measures of genital arousal in women include vaginal photoplethysmography, clitoral ultrasonography, heated oxygen electrode, vaginal thermistor, labial thermistor clip, thermal imaging, and magnetic reso-nance imaging. Although these measures have been used in research settings, their clinical utility is constrained by the necessity of sexual arousal induction, equipment, trained technicians, and interpretive problems. It is interesting to note that these limitations have not hampered the clinical use of similar tech-niques in the clinical assessment of male erectile dysfunction (Levin, 2004).

Psychological Treatment
There have been no RCTs for the psychological treatment of FSAD. This may in part be attributable to the rarity of cases in which FSAD is not secondary to low desire. This clinical reality supports the proposed combination of arousal and desire problems into one new category in the upcoming version of the DSM. On the other hand, the treatment outcome literature for HSDD is not that much better. In any case, the psychological treatment for sexual arousal prob-lems generally focuses on sensate focus and on directed masturbation (Brotto et al., 2010). A number of other interventions included in the generic template are designed to improve the competence of stimulation, and they would also be recommended (e.g., optimizing time and context, use of erotica and sexual aids, sexual imagery and fantasy, and romantic activation).

Hormone Treatment
Administered to women who are androgen-deficient, testosterone has been found to have a beneficial effect on genital arousal as measured by genital vasocongestion (Tuiten et al., 1996). There is also evidence that vaginal appli-cation of dehydroepiandrosterone (DHEA) has quick effects on vaginal tissue and improved sexual desire, arousal, and dyspareunia. Estrogen, locally and systemically administered, has been found to improve vaginal atrophy, vaginal dryness, and physical discomfort with intercourse (Brotto et al., 2010). The main concern with all of these treatments relates to the possible adverse effects of producing supraphysiological levels of hormones in women. Safety data on these interventions are insufficient. In addition, even when genital arousal is increased, there is little evidence that this is accompanied by increases in subjective arousal. Ultimately, it is the latter that is most closely related to women's pleasure and satisfaction.

Nonhormonal Treatment
The success of the phosphodiesterase-5 inhibitors (PDE-5 inhibitor; e.g., silde-nafil/Viagra) in the treatment of arousal problems in men has led to a number of clinical trials investigating the effect of PDE-5 inhibitors on female sexual arousal. Vasocongestion, however, does not appear to be as central to female sexual arousal as it is to male sexual arousal. The results from these studies are mixed, at best. A common report is that these medications have little impact on subjective sexual arousal or subjective perception of increased genital arousal. Results are also mixed for other vasoactive agents such as alprostadil and phentolamine. As such, there is currently no approved vasoactive medication for the treatment of FSAD (Brotto et al., 2010).

Female Orgasmic Disorder

Assessment

Women with acquired female orgasmic disorder (FOD) will quite simply report in a clinical interview that they have either stopped having orgasms, have more difficulty attaining them, or that the intensity of their orgasms has diminished. Women with lifelong orgasmic difficulty will typically report never having had an orgasm, not being sure if they have ever had one, or not understanding what all the fuss is about as they do not feel the kind of pleasure with orgasm everyone else is alluding to. Because orgasm is more of a discrete event than arousal or desire, the assessment of FOD tends to be more straightforward.

There is no self-administered measure specific to FOD. All measures of global sexual function (see Table 5), however, inquire directly about orgasm. Although these measures can be helpful in indicating a potential problem, the questions embedded in these global sexual function questionnaires are not sufficient to establish a nuanced clinical picture of the many variations possible in female orgasmic difficulty. The clinical interview is the best assessment tool for that purpose. Measures of global sexual function will, however, be useful in identifying comorbid sexual dysfunctions. Lack of arousal and desire are common in women who present with FOD.

It is also recommended that an assessment be made as to whether the orgasm difficulty might be secondary to biomedical factors. SSRIs are of particular relevance to FOD as they have been consistently found to interfere with orgasm in women. Conditions involving nerve damage and abdominal surgeries are other potential physiological complications to investigate during the intake.

Psychological Treatment

Because of the high comorbidity among FOD, HSDD, and FSAD, it can be difficult to tease apart the treatment outcome studies for these sexual dysfunctions. Often, studies that bill themselves as targeting one of these dysfunctions are really targeting disturbances at all three stages of sexual response. Perhaps the most distinctive aspect of the treatment of FOD is its focus on the individual woman rather than on the couple, at least in the early stages of treatment.

The guiding principles in the treatment of FOD are the promotion of sex-positive thoughts and attitudes, decreasing anxiety, and increasing the competence of sexual stimuli so as to facilitate orgasm. Education, genital self-exploration, and directed masturbation are particularly germane to the treatment of the woman with lifelong FOD. The literature reports success rates of 80–90% with the use of directed masturbation in the treatment of women with lifelong anorgasmia. Success rates for women with acquired anorgasmia are more varied, with a range from 10% to 75% (Heiman, 2007). The general principle is to instruct the woman in her own sexual stimulation.

Bibliotherapy can be a particularly useful adjunct (see Section 6). The knowledge and skills acquired can then ideally be transferred to partnered sex. It is at this point that the partner becomes more involved in the treatment as either he or she is now instructed in the type of stimulation that works or the client finds ways of self-stimulating in the context of partnered sex. Clearly, any intervention likely to increase arousal (e.g., sensate focus, use of erotica and sex aids and especially vibrators) will be helpful here.

Focusing on relationship dynamics might be particularly indicated if the woman is orgasmic with solitary masturbation but not with a partner. It is important, however, to remind clients that orgasm during partnered sex does not necessarily mean orgasm through intercourse, as a majority of women will likely never or rarely reach orgasm through intercourse alone. On the other hand, couples can be instructed to maximize clitoral stimulation during intercourse. Orgasm through intercourse alone should be no more a goal than simultaneous orgasm. Both set up false expectations for many women and can be damaging to couples.

> **Treatment will vary depending on whether the client is anorgasmic with both masturbation and partnered sex or with partnered sex alone**

Medications

There are currently no approved medications for the treatment of FOD. Testosterone has shown some beneficial effects on orgasm in postmenopausal women (probably mostly through its impact on desire and arousal). However, this type of pharmacological therapy is not without risks. If the woman is taking SSRIs, experimenting with antidepressants that target norepinephrine and dopamine might be useful (e.g., bupropion), as the sexual side effects appear to be lower with these drugs. Vasoactive agents such as sildenafil have not show consistent effects on orgasmic capacity across studies, although some positive outcomes have been reported.

Medical Devices

There are a number of devices that use either suction or electrical stimulation to facilitate orgasm. The Eros Clitoral Therapy Device (Eros CTD) is the only medical device approved for the treatment of FOD. It involves the application of a gentle vacuum to the clitoris to increase blood flow. Slightest Touch is a battery-operated device that stimulates nerve pathways to the genital area by applying electrode pads to the top of the foot and above the ankles and buttocks. These are just two of the devices available, but few women are enthusiastic about these treatments, and most are not rushing out to acquire these devices (for a review, see Ishak, Bokarious, Jeffrey, Davis, & Bakhta, 2010).

Herbal Treatments

There are a number of over-the-counter herbal-based products that claim to impact arousal and orgasmic capacity, including Zestra (a topical botanical massage oil) and ArginMax (a mixture of various herbs and minerals including L-arginine, ginseng, and ginkgo biloba). Limited research indicates that these products may have some impact on arousal and orgasm for some women. Additional research is needed to determine the efficacy of such products, but they are unlikely to be harmful, and trying them generally involves little cost or risk.

Dyspareunia

Assessment

In addition to the integrated multidimensional assessment recommended for all female sexual dysfunctions, the effective assessment of dyspareunia requires specific attention to the properties, potential physical etiology, and functional profile of the pain experienced. A number of self-administered global sexual function measures, such as the SFQ, Female Sexual Function Index (FSFI), Golombok-Rust Inventory of Sexual Satisfaction (GRISS), McCoy Female Sexuality Questionnaire (MFSQ), and the Brief Index of Sexual Functioning for Women (BISF-W), all contain at least one question about pain with intercourse (see Table 5). The only questionnaire focused exclusively on problematic vaginal penetration is the Vaginal Penetration Cognition Questionnaire (VPCQ; Klaassen & ter Kuile, 2009). The VPCQ measures maladaptive cognitions about intercourse, including concerns about control, genital incompatibility, and self-image. It has been found to distinguish between women with dyspareunia and women with vaginismus.

Useful self-administered pain measures include the McGill Pain Questionnaire (MPQ; Melzack, 1975) and the Pain Catastrophizing Scale (PCS; Sullivan, Bishop, & Pivik, 1995), as well as visual analog scales and pain diaries. None of these pain measures, however, will be as useful in locating the pain and investigating its properties as a physical examination. It is essential that the client presenting with dyspareunia be referred to a gynecologist who can attempt to replicate the pain experienced with intercourse via a cotton-swab palpation of the vulva and a pelvic examination. Pukall, Binik, and Khalife (2004) recently introduced an instrument called the vulvalgesiometer to standardize palpation pressure. The palpation serves both to locate the pain precisely and establish the sensitivity of the hyperalgesic area, if one is identified. Assessment of vulvar or pelvic diseases is another important goal of medical referral. Finally, it is also recommended that the client be referred to a physical therapist specializing in pelvic floor dysfunction, as pelvic floor tonicity has been implicated in many cases of dyspareunia (Reissing, Brown, Lord, Binik, & Khalife, 2005).

> The most useful assessment tool in dyspareunia is a pelvic examination with cotton-swab palpation of the vulva

Psychological Treatment

The last 15 years have seen a renaissance in treatment outcome studies for dyspareunia, although most of the research has centered on a specific subtype of dyspareunia, PVD. This is hardly surprising as it is considered to be the most prevalent type of dyspareunia in premenopausal women. Of the nine existing RCTs on dyspareunia, five have examined the impact of CBT and found modest results (ter Kuile, Both, & van Lankveld, 2010).

Although virtually all the generic template treatment components could conceivably be helpful in the treatment of dyspareunia, this dysfunction is unique in its involvement of pain, often excruciating pain. Pain reduction or control usually requires some additional pain-targeted techniques. To date, CBT for dyspareunia has focused on education about the multifactorial nature of both sexual function and pain, cognitive restructuring, rehearsal of coping self-statements, distraction and imagery, relaxation (progressive muscle and breathing), and communication skills training. However, there are a number of behavioral interventions fairly specific to the treatment of dyspareunia (and, as we shall see shortly, vaginismus).

> Group CBT utilizing pain management can be effective in the treatment of PVD

Vaginal dilatation is one such intervention. It basically consists of an in vivo desensitization procedure whereby a woman, in the privacy of her home, inserts a graduated set of dilators over time, making sure that she feels comfortable and relaxed with one size before proceeding to a larger one. "Dilators" is actually a misnomer as there is no dilation involved, but rather a gradual habituation to penetration and a gradual reduction in the involuntary, protective musculature contraction. They do, however, continue to be called dilators, and they can be purchased from various medical suppliers or other sexual aid sources (which are easy to find on the Internet). As the woman moves from beyond her own insertion of the dilators to penile insertion, it is particularly important that she initially control the rate, depth, and movement of those first penile penetration attempts.

Kegel exercises, which involve the repetitive contracting of pelvic floor muscles, have also been used in treatment for dyspareunia to strengthen the pelvic floor as well as to give women a sense of control over their genitalia. Biofeedback electromyography (EMG) with visual feedback has been found to be beneficial. Glazer et al. (1995) trained women to control their pelvic muscle tension in a clinic, using biofeedback. They then completed a pelvic floor training program at home with good results.

Physical Therapy
There are now data to support that pelvic floor tonicity plays a significant role in many cases of dyspareunia and that physical therapy (including education about musculature, manual therapy, biofeedback, electrical stimulation, and home exercises) is an important treatment component (Rosenbaum & Owens, 2008). The national database of the American Physical Therapy Association (http://www.apta.org) lists therapists by location and specialty (e.g., pelvic floor). While vaginal dilatation and Kegel exercises have traditionally been prescribed by psychologists and sex therapists, it is optimal for them to be conducted under the supervision of a pelvic floor physical therapist, as these exercises can be counterproductive in certain cases, depending on the woman's muscular profile and problem.

Medical Treatment
Aside from the medical/surgical treatment of disease states that can produce pain with intercourse (e.g., endometriosis), PVD is the only type of dyspareunia to which medical treatments have been applied. These have included topical analgesic creams, antidepressants (amitriptyline), systemic antifungal (fluconazole) and antiseizure agents (carbamazepine), local corticosteroids, lidocaine, and Botox injections (Landry, Bergeron, Dupuis, & Desrochers, 2008; Petersen, Giraldi, Lundvall, & Kristensen, 2009). Large placebo effects and other methodological difficulties preclude strong support for any one of these strategies, but some appear to work for some women. Referral to a gynecologist with a specialty or interest in vulvar pain disorders is recommended. When pain is unremitting, all reasonable strategies should be thoughtfully considered.

Surgery
This most invasive of treatment strategies is generally indicated only when the dyspareunia has been diagnosed to be PVD and when medical approaches and/or CBT have failed. The surgery of choice is a vestibulectomy, which consists of the excision of the posterior hymen and painful mucosa in the posterior and

anterior vestibule, with or without vaginal mucosa advancement. Although not considered a first line of treatment because of its invasiveness, vestibulectomy boasts more treatment success in both retrospective and prospective studies than any other type of treatment for PVD (Landry et al., 2008). In one RCT that pitted surgery against biofeedback and group CBT, pain reduction was twice as high for participants in the surgery condition than in either of the other two conditions (Bergeron et al., 2001). Long-term follow-up data from this study, however, indicate that CBT may catch up to surgery over time. Additionally, CBT carries little risk, while in the aforementioned study, surgery had resulted in 9% of women reporting a worsening of their pain (Bergeron, Khalife, Glazer, & Binik, 2008).

If a client with PVD has decided to opt for surgery at a given point, she should be encouraged to have a serious discussion with a surgeon about the risks and benefits. She should also be directed to resources to ensure that she is making a truly informed decision.

Alternative Treatments

The research on alternative treatments is not sufficiently rigorous to recommend any particular strategy, but some success has been reported with a hypoallergenic vulvar hygiene program, acupuncture, and hypnosis.

Vaginismus

Assessment

Typically, the diagnosis of vaginismus itself will require little more than the self-report of a woman perceiving full vaginal penetration to be very difficult, if not impossible. Usually, anxiety about penetration is palpable, and there is also a history of difficulty with gynecological examinations. Many will report pain with intercourse attempts. Avoidance of both intercourse and pelvic examinations is high in women with vaginismus.

The assessment of vaginismus does not differ substantially from the assessment of dyspareunia. Both involve difficulty with intercourse, and teasing them apart can sometimes be a challenge. There do, however, appear to be differences between the two populations. On the VPCQ, women with vaginismus report more cognitions related to lack of control, pain catastrophizing, negative self-image, and genital incompatibility than do women with dyspareunia. Anxiety, fear of penetration, and fear of pain are likely to be prominent in cases of vaginismus. Unlike dyspareunia, vaginismus has a phobic-like quality. Because of this, it is a good idea to also assess for other types of anxiety that might be at play.

Although a gynecological/pelvic examination is an important assessment component, it might be initially impossible for some clients, as many cannot tolerate a pelvic exam. In many cases, the physical examination is only possible after psychological treatment has rendered such examinations tolerable. If eventually possible, it is recommended that a pelvic examination be undergone to assess for conditions that might impact the vaginismus or simply for the purpose of maintaining general health (e.g., regular Papanicolaou tests ["Pap smears"]). It is crucial, however, that a gynecologist sensitive to these difficulties be chosen. A negative experience could retraumatize the client and set her back significantly. To ensure as positive an experience as possible, the gynecologist needs to be informed ahead of time that the woman has vaginismus and that a longer block of time needs to be reserved for the examination. It is also important that the patient know in advance exactly what will be attempted and that she be assured full control over the situation (this will likely also be indicated in the examination of women with severe dyspareunia). Referral to a physical therapist for assessment of pelvic floor disturbances is also recommended. Again, this referral needs to be aligned with the client's ability to tolerate such examinations and with a physical therapist who specializes in such cases.

Psychological Treatment

In addition to the broader psychoeducational, cognitive-behavioral, and relational components of therapy for female sexual dysfunctions, systematic desensitization has been the hallmark of treatment for vaginismus. The vaginistic reaction is considered a conditioned fear response to sexual stimuli or other forms of vaginal penetration (as in a gynecological examination). Vaginal dilatation, Kegel exercises, and sensate focus feature prominently in this approach. However, much as with the other sexual dysfunctions, empirical evidence for this treatment strategy is scarce. Only four RCTs investigating the effect of the aforementioned behavioral and CBT approaches have been published (ter Kuile et al., 2010). However, the success rates in these and in uncontrolled studies are relatively high, supporting both the focus on exposure therapy as well as the intense involvement of the therapist in guiding the treatment.

Other Treatments

Depending on how strongly linked the vaginismus is to a more generalized anxiety, SSRIs might be worth trying, although there are no studies specifically testing their efficacy in the treatment of vaginismus. Physical therapy, as tolerated, can also be helpful to address the pelvic floor hypertonicity that is likely implicated in vaginismus.

4.2.   Problems in Carrying Out Treatments

4.2.1   Defining Treatment Success

In part because of the complexity and expansiveness of most cases of female sexual dysfunction, identifying appropriate outcome measures is a challenge to both research and clinical practice. Frequency of sex is often used as a behavioral measure of progress. More sex is interpreted to signal more desire, arousal, and orgasms, as well as less pain. However, *therapy can be effective in changing behavior without necessarily making it a positive experience.* In some nonsexual problems, the movement from aversion to tolerance would be considered a success (e.g., fear of flying). That is rarely the case with sex. Consequently, the outcome that makes the most sense is sexual and emotional satisfaction and pleasure, independent of the frequency or nature of the sexual activity. Most women would be unlikely to proclaim that frequent boring or irritating or painful sex was a treatment success.

Having asserted the primacy of physical and emotional satisfaction as the ultimate goal of therapy for women with sexual problems, some backtracking is warranted. Ultimately, it is the client who gets to decide what treatment success looks like. They decide what kind of sex is good enough and what kind of relationship is worth keeping. This can sometimes be difficult for therapists who start the treatment with their own sexual scripts and definitions of success. Even the seemingly universal goal of satisfaction heralded in the previous paragraph may not generalize to everyone. For example, the therapist confronted with a woman with vaginismus who just wants to be able to have a baby and seems unconcerned with pleasure or satisfaction may find this challenging as it goes against our 21st-century, secular, and Western sexual script (see Section 4.3 "Multicultural Issues," below). The bottom line is, however, that therapists do not get to decide what clients want.

Furthermore, there are few fantasy endings in the treatment of sexual problems. As we have reviewed in this text, sexuality is dizzyingly multidimensional, and disturbances in sexual function and relationships often have long developmental pasts. Disabusing clients of unreasonable expectations (often propagated by unattainable media ideals), while still maintaining hope and the drive to achieve as much as possible, is a challenge. However, sometimes the bigger challenge can be for therapists to drop their own sexual and relationship ideals and accept it when clients claim that they are happy with a level of progress that the therapist finds disappointing.

4.2.2   Sex as Homework

Homework assignments centered on cognitive restructuring and behavioral activation are a central component of CBT. Compliance with these assignments is, however, hardly guaranteed. Clients can fail to buy into the treatment rationale, feeling that it simplifies a complex problem. Therapists can lack skill in the instruction, review, and reinforcement of assignments. At the most basic level, it is natural that clients will have a natural resistance to start doing what they have been avoiding or never even tried.

Positioning sexual activity as "homework" can be problematic

Sex, however, adds an extra complication. Sex is supposed to be fun and not another item on the to-do list. The therapist and client can thus find themselves in the paradoxical situation of having to promote or do "work" to have fun. In addition, these assignments will go counter to the spontaneity script of sex. If one is to engage in CBT for sexual problems, there is no way to avoid the suspension of the spontaneity script, at least temporarily. When sex is not happening and/or pleasure is not forthcoming when it does, most couples will agree with the therapist that "spontaneity" may need some nudging. This is a helpful discussion to have before starting the assignments. A detail that can help is to use language judiciously when speaking of these assignments. The word *homework* is probably best left out. Asking directly about the activity assigned is preferable (e.g., "how did things go with the sensual massage?" rather than "how did the homework assignment go?").

4.2.3 Negotiating the Level of Structure

A discussion about the desired level of structure in the treatment is recommended. Some couples will want to leave each session with a scheduled date for their sensate focus assignment or for their romantic evening and an agreement on who will initiate the activity. Others will find this mechanistic, "fake," and counterproductive. The latter may commit to an assignment but prefer to leave some spontaneity intact. Letting clients express their preference for structure is a good idea at the beginning. The level of structure can then be adjusted depending on its success. The initially structure-loving couple may eventually feel a little too stifled by the schedule, while the more free-wheeling couple may discover that a failure to schedule leads to either nonaction or disappointment in a partner's perceived lack of initiative.

4.2.4 Avoiding Therapist-Induced Performance Anxiety

One of the paradoxes of directive interventions for sexual problems is that the therapist can unwittingly find himself/herself in the position of exerting pressure on the client to engage in sexual activity. *This must be avoided at all costs.* The performance anxiety that many clients already have should certainly not be compounded by the therapist. Avoiding this pitfall involves the in-depth discussion of nonadherence to assignments or directives, and the constant reminder, verbally and behaviorally, that the client is in control of the pace of therapy and free to make choices. The discussion of her choices, especially when they involve continued avoidance of sexual activity, should be characterized by openness and a desire for understanding rather than by the pathologizing of the avoidance. The woman gets to want what she wants, without shame or pressure from a therapist. If she wants to change, then the treatment can proceed through planned stages. If she does not, then the therapist can help her understand and own her choice.

> **Perceived pressure from the therapist can create another layer of performance anxiety**

4.2.5 Attention to Secondary Gain

Because most people consider sex an intensely pleasurable activity, it can be difficult, even for therapists, to imagine sexual dysfunctions delivering any benefits. However, they often do, and the secondary gain may be experienced by the woman and/or her partner. The most common secondary gain within the couple system is the maintenance of the couple's stability. For example, one person's sexual dysfunction may be alleviating the insecurity of the other. The sexual dysfunction may be abating fears of abandonment or infidelity in the more insecure partner. Alternately, a partner with low desire may unconsciously feel a sense of control in her doling out of sex – a control that she does not feel in the nonsexual aspects of her relationship. It is not uncommon for sexual dynamics to mirror relationship dynamics, and there are many potential variations of secondary gain in sexual dysfunction.

The most obvious way in which the secondary gain reveals itself in therapy is when one or both members of the couple do not appear as happy as you might have predicted when real treatment gains are made (e.g., a husband complaining about his wife's sexual technique in their first sexual episode after an entirely sexless year; a woman unenthusiastically reporting she had no pain during intercourse for the first time in months). Typically, clients are not conscious of secondary gains and can be defensive when confronted with such an interpretation of events or of their affect. One way to approach secondary gain concerns is to integrate them into the clinical interview as shown below. However, it is often much later that clients discover that the sexual dysfunction may serve some secondary purpose, despite the primary losses it predominantly represents. Below are some questions to ask both members of the couple so as to investigate the possibility of secondary gain:

(1) How do you think your life would change if you (or your partner) had more sexual desire / more arousal / more orgasms / less pain?
(2) Are there any ways in which more sexual desire / more arousal / more orgasms / less pain might complicate things for you (or your partner)?
(3) Make a list of the pros and cons of having this problem.
(4) Do you have any worries about treatment for this problem and what it might uncover?

This type of exploration has much in common with motivational interviewing and can reveal some system-embedded barriers to change.

4.3 Multicultural Issues

4.3.1 Gender

The historically consistent script for female sexuality has largely been low sexual agency and high sexual objectification

There is probably no aspect of life more gender-differentiated than sexuality. Cultures vary on many dimensions but gender-differentiated norms for the sexual behavior of women and men are close to universal. Generally speaking, the near universal code for the desired behavior of women is characterized by low sexual agency and high sexual objectification. These norms have an impact on female clients, their partners, and their therapists. This is particularly true in the case of therapy for sexual dysfunction, the very definition of which is likely to reflect and often reinforce these norms (e.g., women who have pain with intercourse have a sexual problem rather than a pain problem).

No one therapist is a match for centuries-old, ubiquitous societal norms, no matter how harmful some may be. However, making clients aware that these ideas are adopted cultural values rather than inevitabilities can help free some female clients to assert what they want and what they do not want in therapy and with their partner. Some clients will feel no tension with gendered cultural values, while others will rail against them. As with any other set of cultural beliefs, the therapist needs to respect the position of the client, while educating them and helping them reach their goals in as value-free a way as possible.

4.3.2 Religious and Cultural Norms

Over and above the question of gender, clients will come into therapy with varying religious beliefs and cultural norms. Some clients' belief systems will be what Western therapists consider "sex-positive," while others will take a stance to sex that is more prohibitive and centered on reproduction rather than pleasure. Clearly, sex therapy is a Western phenomenon that assumes the primacy of pleasure, promotes a diversity of sexual stimuli and activities, and assigns masturbation and vaginal dilatation exercises liberally in the treatment of dysfunctions. It is not difficult to imagine how many of these techniques might be in direct conflict with certain cultural and religious values. To help as many people as possible, psychotherapy for sexual problems cannot position itself outside of the range of all cultures other than Western and/or secular ones.

Exploring the religious or cultural beliefs of clients who present with sexual difficulties is an important component of the clinical interview (See Appendices 2 and 3). It will inform the therapist about what types of interventions are likely to be acceptable to the client. Well after the initial clinical interview, it is still recommended that the introduction of any technique or intervention first be vetted by the client for cultural/religious acceptability. Therapists cannot be expected to know the details of every client's culture or religion, but they can ask the client to educate them and let them know when a technique is not acceptable to them. Failing to do so can lead to an early dropout. An example with a case of vaginismus would be as follows:

Therapist: Over the years, doctors in our field have found that it is helpful for women with your problem to start inserting vaginal dilators of increasing size until the woman is comfortable with the insertion of a dilator that approaches the size of her husband's penis [this may have to be explained in more detail or using different words]. I am aware of the fact that this may seem like an unusual treatment, but we have had success with it, and we think it may help you and your husband. How do you and your husband feel about starting this type of treatment? I need to know from you whether there is anything about this treatment that you feel goes against your beliefs. If it does, that's OK, we can try other strategies.

Often, when the intervention is positioned as a treatment rather than as a pleasure-inducing activity, even very conservative clients will find it palatable. They need to be able to distinguish "treatment" from what might be perceived as erotica.

Being culturally competent when treating women from diverse cultures thus requires adherence to four basic principles: (1) be aware that you, the therapist, are no less attached to a set of values about sexuality than any of your clients; (2) become educated in your client's values and beliefs (via your clients themselves and via external sources); (3) vet all interventions/techniques by your client's values; and (4) be flexible in adapting interventions to clients' belief systems.

4.3.3   Sexual Identity and Orientation

The predominantly male and Western-identified culture from which therapy for sexual problems arises also has another attribute; it is hetero-centrist.

The vast majority of published research and clinical reports emanate from heterosexual populations. Consequently, we have little information about the treatment of sexual difficulties in gay, lesbian, bisexual, and transgendered individuals. Many of the principles and interventions covered in this book are likely to be relevant to the treatment of bisexual women, lesbians, and trans-women. One should not assume that their difficulty is rooted in sexual identity and/or orientation. On the other hand, the competent therapist is aware of potential additional issues that may need to be attended to.

On the negative side, the social stigmatization of these groups of women may surface in their sexual function and relationships. On the positive side, sexual practices may be more varied and diverse than most therapists know, and their openness to change greater than in the heterosexual client. The therapist needs to be educated about the histories of such clients, both developmental and social/societal. Yet again, clients are our best sources of education. An honest, direct request for them to educate us about certain aspects of their lives is usually positively responded to and can strengthen rapport. This does not, of course, preclude our own research and reading of relevant materials. Most importantly, therapists need to drop their own sexual scripts about normality, gender, relationships, and acceptable erotic practices (Nichols & Shernoff, 2007).

5

Case Vignette

The case described below is a complicated one involving HSDD (with features of SAD) and FOD. It highlights the comorbidity of female sexual dysfunctions, the primacy of relationship concerns, and the ambiguity of treatment outcome success.

Kristina was a married, 35-year-old musician who first presented alone, requesting therapy for low sexual desire. She had been married to 36-year-old Kevin for 10 years, whom she described as "reasonably attractive" and a loving husband. They had no children. She, however, could not care less if they ever had sex again. She reported that, at the start of the relationship, she was very attracted to him and sexually desirous, but that this had quickly faded and been replaced by a "roommate" kind of relationship. Kristina would grudgingly comply with his sexual requests once a month out of guilt. Aside from her concern that her sexual avoidance was upsetting him, she was also wondering whether there was something wrong with her.

In the clinical interview she reported having had desire for partners prior to Kevin, but that it was usually strongest for the type of "bad boy" that she knew would make a terrible husband and father. When speaking of sex, her facial expressions communicated a certain level of distaste approaching disgust. When asked about orgasms, she claimed to not be sure whether she had ever had one. Kristina described sensations during sex that sounded very much like arousal, but at a certain intensity level, she would abruptly push him off because the sensations became "too much." She had never masturbated, and she had never let anyone perform oral sex on her (the thought of the latter disgusted her). She did not have pain with intercourse, and she seemed mostly distressed about the impact of her lack of desire on Kevin and her musings about whether Kevin was exciting enough for her.

The clinical interview did not indicate any physical problems, and she reported having recently undergone a full work-up with her family physician, including an endocrine panel. All had come up normal. There was no history of abuse or trauma, and her psychosocial history seemed unremarkable in relation to sexual dysfunction risk factors. After asserting that her goal for therapy was to increase her sexual desire, it was recommended that Kevin join her in treatment, which he willingly did. The intake with Kevin revealed no sexual dysfunction on his part and another unremarkable risk factor profile.

Sessions 1–3 were devoted to education about desire, arousal and orgasm, and an assessment of their relationship dynamics in sexual and nonsexual domains. The couple was clearly stuck in two variations of the demand–withdrawal pattern. In regards to sex, he was the one making demands, and she was the one withdrawing. The more he requested sex and the more he complained about them not having it, the less likely she was to give in. In the nonsexual realm, she was the one making demands – on his time, on his attention, on work around the house – and the more she did this, the more he would go out with his friends or retreat to the room he called his "man cave." Their relationship history revealed that Kristina had given up the pursuit of a music career to marry Kevin and follow him to another city where he had secured employment. She had become a music teacher and always wondered if she could have made it as a professional musician, had she stuck to her career plans instead of opting to follow Kevin.

Kevin and Kristina were also asked to stop trying to have sex until indicated by the therapist who would instruct them on how to go about it in different ways. The point here was to disrupt their maladaptive sexual patterns and eventually reset them.

Sessions 4–9 were simultaneously focused on optimizing arousal and on relationship skills building. In Session 4, the couple was introduced to sensate focus, and they were given their first assignment of nondemand, nongenital pleasuring followed by mutual corrective feedback. Kristina was also assigned a genital self-exploration exercise. They were both asked to track their thoughts about their sexual and nonsexual relationship interactions, if and when these resulted in any distress. Sessions 5–10 consisted of a gradual progression through cognitive restructuring, sensate focus, and directed masturbation exercises (the latter just for Kristina). During these exercises, it became evident that Kristina's low desire involved a certain degree of sexual aversion, although anxiety did not feature prominently.

Their conflicting sexual scripts quickly became apparent. Kristina was stuck in a dichotomous "sex versus love" view of relationships wherein sex was a bad, naughty thing that you only enjoyed with people you did not love and who did not love you (hence her attraction to "bad boys"). In contrast, Kevin approached sex as an unremarkable bodily need that could mercifully be satisfied within a loving relationship. Neither sexual script was conducive to satisfying sex.

This stage of therapy intensely targeted their relationship. In addition to romantic activation and communication skills training, the couple was introduced to the concept of differentiation and asked to track ways in which they owned or failed to own their choices, thoughts, and emotions. For the first time, both Kristina and Kevin saw how they were both putting far more responsibility for their individual well-being on their partners than was reasonable. Their sexual scripts were also analyzed for maladaptive relationship beliefs. Some of these scripts related to gendered notions of marriage and careers.

By Session 11, Kristina and Kevin started having sex. There was excellent progress on some fronts and less in others. Genital self-exploration was no longer uncomfortable for Kristina, and her feelings of disgust had abated significantly. The directed masturbation, however, had failed to result in orgasm. She continued to report high arousal but no culmination. She was instructed to continue stimulating herself past the point at which she had initially reported needing to stop, but it had not worked. She reported that her arousal simply went away at that point. It almost sounded like an orgasm but without the associated intense pleasure. Not surprisingly, she also remained anorgasmic with partnered sex. However, the sensate focus exercises had been successful in vastly improving the quality of their sexual interactions, and both Kristina and Kevin reported more arousal than they had felt in a long time.

As to feelings of sexual desire, Kristina reported that she still never felt spontaneous desire. However, when Kevin initiated or when she decided to initiate, the desire would start once she started to feel aroused by the stimulation. She remained disappointed about her inability to orgasm but was pleased with the improvements. The most dramatic turnaround was in the nature of their relationship. The therapy appeared to have effected a paradigm shift, and both of them reported that they felt they were "in a different relationship" – a much better one. Session 12 was focused on ways to identify the possible return of concerning patterns of thoughts, emotions, and behaviors, and how to target them before they became entrenched.

Two years later, they returned for four booster sessions. Two major positive life events were having a negative impact on their sex. Kristina had successfully reentered the professional music scene, but this left her with less time and flexibility than before. This was compounded by the birth of their daughter, which had also disrupted their new, more positive sexual and nonsexual dynamic. Being a mother had re-reactivated Kristina's old sexual script, and she felt an incompatibility between her "mother persona" and her "sexual persona." Despite Kevin's initial encouragement of Kristina's return to music, he was feeling threatened by her new career and jealous of her attention to their little girl. While acknowledging the inevitable changes that busy professional lives and parenting will have on a romantic relationship, the four sessions focused on (1) the renewed deconstruction of their respective scripts negatively impacting the relationship, and (2) brainstorming specific ways to adapt to their new context without losing their love/sex story.

6

Further Reading

Selected Readings for Professionals

Goldstein, A. T., Pukall, C. F., & Goldstein, I. (Eds.). (2009). *Female sexual pain disorders*. Oxford: Wiley-Blackwell.

A scholarly and clinically practical collection of chapters by the leading experts on multiple aspects and types of sexual pain.

Hertlein, K. M., Weeks, G. R., & Gambescia, N. (Eds.). (2009). *Systemic sex therapy*. New York: Routledge

A user-friendly introduction to sex therapy from a systems perspective for the graduate student or the generalist seeking to self-educate in the treatment of sexual problems. A clinician's guide is also available.

Leiblum, S. R. (Ed.). (2007). *Principles and practice of sex therapy* (4th ed.). New York: Guilford Press.

Often considered the top reference text for sex therapy, this is an invaluable resource for clinicians. Look out for the soon-to-be-published fifth edition by new editors Y. M. Binik and K. Hall.

Leiblum, S. R. (Ed.). (2010). *Treating sexual desire disorders: A clinical case book*. New York: Guilford.

Focused on the most common sexual dysfunction, this clinical case book covers a wide range of approaches to the treatment of real cases of HSDD.

Levine, S. B. (Ed.). (2010). *Handbook of clinical sexuality for mental health professionals*. New York: Routledge.

This highly readable edited book is written specifically for mental health professionals without an established expertise in sex therapy.

Maurice, W. L. (1999). *Sexual medicine in primary care*. New York: Mosby.

Although no longer in press, the entire book is downloadable for free at http://www.kinseyinstitute.org. It provides excellent guidelines for diagnostic interviewing for sexual difficulties.

Schnarch, D. M. (1991). *Constructing the sexual crucible: An integration of sexual and marital therapy*. New York: W. W. Norton.

Theoretically situated in attachment theory, this monograph remains an important contribution to integrative sex and marital therapy with its whole relationship approach to sexual problems. Written over 20 years ago, it remains fresh.

Wincze, J. P. (2009). *Enhancing sexuality: A problem-solving approach to treating dysfunction. Therapist guide*. New York: Oxford University Press.

A pragmatic guide to the treatment of sexual problems. The workbook for clients is particularly useful, especially for the clinician first starting out in this area.

Selected Readings for Consumers

Barbach, L. (2000). *For yourself: The fulfillment of female sexuality*. New York: Signet.

This classic text empowers and guides women to discover their own sexuality in a compassionate manner. An excellent read for women with difficulties or just questions about their sexuality.

Goldstein, A. T., & Brandon, M. (2009). *Reclaiming desire: Four keys to finding your lost libido*. New York: Rodale Books.

A practical guide to problems of low desire, this book investigates the many factors that interfere with women's desire focusing on physical health, emotional resilience, intellectual fulfillment, and spiritual contentment.

Goldstein, A. T., Pukall, C. F., & Goldstein, I. (2011). *When sex hurts: A woman's guide to banishing pain*. New York: Da Capo Lifelong Books.

This is a welcome text for any woman experiencing pain with sex. It skillfully validates the woman's experience while considering all the possible causes and available treatments.

Hall, K. (2004). *Reclaiming your sexual self: How to bring desire back into your life*. New York: Wiley.

This intelligent and warm book takes a holistic approach to women's desire and shares clinical strategies to help women find their way back to their sexuality.

Hanh, T. N. (1999). *The miracle of mindfulness: An introduction to the practice of meditation*. Boston: Beacon Press.

An accessible introduction to the practice of mindfulness meditation.

Heiman, J., & LoPiccolo, J. (1987). *Becoming orgasmic: A sexual and personal growth program for women*. New York: Fireside.

This classic continues to be very effective in laying out a specific strategy for the woman who is anorgasmic or has difficulty enjoying sex.

Herbenick, D. (2009). *Because it feels good: A woman's guide to sexual pleasure and satisfaction*. New York: Rodale.

With its focus on sexual pleasure, this book is part sex education and part empowerment guide for women wanting to explore their sexuality.

Kabat-Zinn, J. (2006). *Mindfulness for beginners* [audio CD]. Louisville, CO: Sounds True Inc.

Very skillful audio CD consisting of guided exercises led by the American master of mindfulness. Probably more effective in teaching mindfulness than a book.

Leiblum, S. R., & Sachs, J. (2003). *Getting the sex you want: A woman's guide to becoming proud, passionate, and pleased in bed*. New York: iUniverse.

With a keen eye toward all of the demands on women's lives, Leiblum suggests ways to navigate the complexities while holding on to and nurturing your sexual self.

McCarthy, B. W., & McCarthy, E. J. (2003). *Rekindling desire: A step-by-step program to help with low-sex and no-sex marriages*. New York: Routledge.

This intimacy focused book gives practical advice to both men and women whose sex lives have suffered setbacks common in long-term relationships.

Ogden, G. (2008). *The return of desire: A guide to rediscovering your sexual passion*. New York: Trumpeter.

In this holistic approach to desire and passion, emphasis is placed on the deeper aspects of our sexual connections and the link between sexuality and spirituality.

Perel, E. (2006). *Mating in captivity: Reconciling the erotic and the domestic*. New York: Harper Collins.

This is a refreshing look at the challenge of maintaining passion in long-term relationships, claiming that intimacy or closeness can sometimes be the culprit.

Schnarch, D. M. (2003). *Resurrecting sex: Solving sexual problems and revolutionizing your relationship*. New York: Harper Paperbacks.

In this book, Schnarch illustrates the ways in which relationship enmeshment can interfere with true intimacy and good sex. A smart book with in-depth analyses of how couples can find their way back to differentiated and healthy connections.

7

References

Althof, S. (2001). My personal distress over the inclusion of personal distress. *Journal of Sex and Marital Therapy, 27,* 123–125.

American Psychiatric Association. (1987). *Diagnostic and statistical manual of mental disorders* (3rd ed., revised). Washington, DC: Author.

American Psychiatric Association. (2000). *Diagnostic and statistical manual of mental disorders* (4th ed., text revision). Washington, DC: Author.

American Psychiatric Association. (2012, March16). *DSM-5 development: Sexual and gender identity disorders.* Retrieved from http://www.dsm5.org

Andersen, B. L., & Cyranowski, J. M. (1994). Women's sexual self-schema. *Journal of Personality and Social Psychology, 67,* 1079–1100.

Apperloo, M. J. A., Van der Stege, J. G., Hoek, A., & Weijmar Schultz, W. C. M. (2003). In the mood for sex: The value of androgens. *Journal of Sex and Marital Therapy, 29,* 87–102.

Apt, C. V., & Hurlbert, D. F. (1992). Motherhood and female sexuality beyond one year postpartum: A study of military wives. *Journal of Sex Education and Therapy, 18,* 104–114.

Ashton, A. K. (2007). The new sexual pharmacology: A guide for the clinician. In S. R. Leiblum (Ed.), *Principles and practice of sex therapy* (4th ed., pp. 509–542). New York: Guilford Press.

Bancroft, J., & Janssen, E. (2000). The dual control model of male sexual response: A theoretical approach to centrally mediated erectile dysfunction. *Neuroscience and Biobehavioral Reviews, 23,* 763–784.

Barlow, D. H. (1986). The causes of sexual dysfunction: The role of anxiety and cognitive interference. *Journal of Consulting and Clinical Psychology, 54,* 140–148.

Basson, R. (2007). Sexual desire/arousal disorders in women. In S. R. Leiblum (Ed.), *Principles and practice of sex therapy* (4th ed., pp. 25–53). New York: Guilford Press.

Baumeister, R. F. (2000). Gender differences in erotic plasticity: The female sex drive as socially flexible and responsive. *Psychological Bulletin, 126,* 347–374.

Baumeister, R. F., Catanese, K., & Vohs, K. (2001). Is there a gender difference in strength of sex drive? Theoretical views, conceptual distinction, and a review of relevant evidence. *Personality and Social Psychology Review, 5,* 242–273.

Bergeron, S., Binik, Y. M., Khalife, S., Pagidas, K., Glazer, H. I., Meana, M., & Amsel, R. (2001). A randomized comparison of group cognitive-behavioral therapy, surface electromyographic biofeedback, and vestibulectomy in the treatment of dyspareunia resulting from vulvar vestibulitis. *Pain, 91,* 297–306.

Bergeron, S., Khalife, S., Glazer, H. I., & Binik, Y. M. (2008). Surgical and behavioral treatments for vestibulodynia: Two-and-one-half year follow-up and predictors of outcome. *Obstetrics and Gynecology, 111,* 159–166.

Binik, Y. M. (2010a). The DSM diagnostic criteria for dyspareunia. *Archives of Sexual Behavior, 39,* 292–303.

Binik, Y. M. (2010b). The DSM diagnostic criteria for vaginismus. *Archives of Sexual Behavior, 39,* 278–291.

Binik, Y. M., & Meana, M. (2009). The future of sex therapy: Specialization or marginalization? *Archives of Sexual Behavior, 38,* 1016–1027.

Both, S., Spiering, M., Everaerd, W., & Laan, E. (2004). Sexual behavior and responsiveness to sexual cues following laboratory-induced sexual arousal. *Journal of Sex Research, 41,* 242–259.

Bradford, A., & Meston, C. M. (2009). Placebo response in the treatment of women's sexual dysfunctions: A review and commentary. *Journal of Sex & Marital Therapy, 35,* 164–181.

Brotto, L. A. (2010). The DSM diagnostic criteria for hypoactive sexual desire disorder in women. *Archives of Sexual Behavior, 39,* 221–239.

Brotto, L. A., Bitzer, J., Laan, E., Leiblum, S., & Luria, M. (2010). Women's sexual desire and arousal disorders. *Journal of Sexual Medicine, 7,* 586–614.

Brotto, L. A., Basson, R., & Luria, M. (2008). A mindfulness-based group psychoeducational intervention targeting sexual arousal disorder in women. *Journal of Sexual Medicine, 5,* 1646–1659.

Brotto, L. A., Heiman, J. R., & Tolman, D. L. (2009). Narratives of desire in mid-age women with and without arousal difficulties. *Journal of Sex Research, 46,* 387–398.

Brotto, L. A., Yule, M., & Breckon, E. (2010). Psychological interventions for the sexual sequelae of cancer: A review of the literature. *Journal of Cancer Survivorship, 4,* 346–360.

Burri, A. V., Cherkas, L. M., & Spector, T. D. (2009). The genetics and epidemiology of female sexual dysfunction: A review. *Journal of Sexual Medicine, 6,* 646–657.

Clayton, A. H., Goldfischer, E. R., Goldstein, I., Derogatis, L., Lewis-D'Agostino, D. J., & Pyke, R. (2009). Validation of the Decreased Sexual Desire Screener (DSDS): A brief diagnostic instrument for generalized acquired female Hypoactive Sexual Desire Disorder (HSDD). *Journal of Sexual Medicine, 6,* 730–738.

Clayton, A. H., Segraves, R. T., Leiblum, S., Basson, R., Pyke, R., Cotton, D., ... Wunderlich, G. R. (2006). Reliability and validity of the Sexual Interest and Desire Inventory-Female (SIDI-F), a scale designed to measure severity of female Hypoactive Sexual Desire Disorder. *Journal of Sex and Marital Therapy, 12,* 115–135.

Clayton, A. H., Warnock, J. K., Kornstein, S. G., Pinkerton, R., Sheldon-Keller, A., & McGarvey, E. L. (2004). A placebo-controlled trial of bupropion SR as an antidote for selective serotonin reuptake inhibitor-induced sexual dysfunction. *Journal of Clinical Psychiatry, 65,* 62–67.

Clement, U. (2002). Sex in long-term relationships: A systematic approach to sexual desire problems. *Archives of Sexual Behavior, 31,* 241–246.

Cyranowski, J. M., Frank, E., Cherry, C., Huck, P., & Kupfer, D. (2004). Prospective assessment of sexual function in women treated for recurrent major depression. *Journal of Psychiatric Research, 38,* 267–273.

Davis, H. J., & Reissing, E. D. (2007). Relationship adjustment and dyadic interaction in couples with sexual pain disorders: A critical review of the literature. *Sexual and Relationship Therapy, 22,* 245–254.

Davis, S. R., Davison, S. L., Donath, S., & Bell, R. J. (2005). Circulating androgen levels and self-reported sexual function in women. *Journal of the American Medical Association, 294,* 91–96.

Dennerstein, L., Koochaki, P., Barton, I., & Graziottin, A. (2006). Hypoactive sexual desire disorder in menopausal women: A survey of western European women. *Journal of Sexual Medicine, 3,* 212–222.

Derogatis, L. R. (1997). The Derogatis Interview for Sexual Functioning (DISF/DISF-SR): An introductory report. *Journal of Sex & Marital Therapy, 23,* 291–304.

Derogatis, L. R., Allgood, A., Eubank, D., Greist, J., Bharmal, M., Zipfel, L., & Guo, C.-Y. (2010). Validation of a women's sexual interest Diagnostic Interview: Short Form (WSID-SF) and a Daily Log of Sexual Activities (DLSA) in postmenopausal women with hypoactive sexual desire disorder. *Journal of Sexual Medicine, 7,* 917–927.

Derogatis, L. R., Rosen, R., Leiblum, S., Burnett, A., & Heiman, J. (2002). The Female Sexual Distress Scale (FSDS): Initial validation of a standardized scale for assessment of sexually related personal distress in women. *Journal of Sex and Marital Therapy, 28,* 317–330.

Derogatis, L. R., Rust, J., Golombok, S., Bouchard, C., Nachtigall, L., Rodenberg, C., ... McHorney, C. A. (2004). Validation of the Profile of Female Sexual Function (PFSF) in surgically and naturally menopausal women. *Journal of Sex and Marital Therapy, 30,* 25–36.

Desrosiers, M., Bergeron, S., Meana, M., Leclerc, B., Binik, Y. M., & Khalife, S. (2008). Psychosexual characteristics of vestibulodynia couples: Partner solicitousness and hostility are associated with pain. *Journal of Sexual Medicine, 5,* 418–427.

Donaldson, R. L., & Meana, M. (2011). Early dyspareunia experience in young women: Confusion, consequences, and help-seeking barriers. *Journal of Sexual Medicine, 8,* 814– 823.

Finch, S. (2001). Sexual Aversion Disorder treated with behavioural desensitization. *The Canadian Journal of Psychiatry, 46,* 563–564.

Fisher, W. A., Byrne, D., White, L. A., & Kelley, K. (1988). Erotophobia-erotophilia as a dimension of personality. *Journal of Sex Research, 25,* 123–151.

Fugl-Meyer, A. R., & Fugl-Meyer, K. S. (1999). Sexual disabilities, problems and satisfaction in 18–74 year old Swedes. *Scandinavian Journal of Sexology, 2,* 79–105.

Glazer, H. I., Rodke, G., Swencionis, C., Hertz, R., & Young, A.W. (1995). The treatment of vulvar vestibulitis syndrome by electromyographic biofeedback of pelvic floor musculature. *Journal of Reproductive Medicine, 40,* 283–290.

Gold, S. R., & Gold, R. G. (1993). Sexual aversions: A hidden disorder. In W. O'Donohue & J. H. Geer (Eds.). *Handbook of sexual dysfunctions: Assessment and treatment* (pp. 83–102). Needham Heights, MA: Allyn & Bacon.

Goldstat, R., Briganti, E., Tran, J., Wolfe, R., & Davis, S. R. (2003). Transdermal testosterone therapy improves well-being, mood, and sexual function in premenopausal women. *Menopause, 10,* 390–98.

Gottman, J. M. (1999). *The marriage clinic.* New York: Norton.

Graham, C. A. (2010a). The DSM diagnostic criteria for female sexual arousal disorder. *Archives of Sexual Behavior, 39,* 240–255

Graham, C. A. (2010b). The DSM diagnostic criteria for female orgasmic disorder. *Archives of Sexual Behavior, 39,* 256–270.

Graham, C. A., Sanders, S. A., Milhausen, R. R., & McBride, K. R. (2004). Turning on and turning off: A focus group study of the factors that affect women's sexual arousal. *Archives of Sexual Behavior, 33,* 527–538.

Granot, M. (2005). Personality traits associated with perception of noxious stimuli in women with vulvar vestibulitis syndrome. *Journal of Pain, 6,* 168–173.

Hall, K. (2007). Sexual dysfunction and childhood sexual abuse: Gender differences and treatment implications. In S. R. Leiblum (Ed.), *Principles and practice of sex therapy* (4th ed., pp. 350–378). New York: Guilford Press.

Harlow, B. L., Wise, L. A., & Stewart, E. G. (2001). Prevalence and predictors of chronic lower genital tract discomfort. *American Journal of Obstetrics and Gynecology, 185,* 545–550.

Hartmann, U., Philippsohn, S., Heiser, K., & Ruffer-Hesse, C. (2004). Low desire in midlife and older women: Personality factors, psychosocial development, present sexuality. *Menopause, 11,* 726–740.

Hawton, K. (1985). *Sex therapy: A practical guide.* Northvale, NJ: Aronson.

Hayes, R. D. (2011). Circular and linear modeling of female sexual desire and arousal. *Journal of Sex Research, 48,* 130–141.

Hayes, R. D., Bennett, C. M., Fairley, C. K., & Dennerstein, L. (2006). What can prevalence studies tells us about female sexual difficulty and dysfunction? *Journal of Sexual Medicine, 3,* 589–595.

Hayes, R. D., & Dennerstein, L. (2005) The impact of aging on sexual function and dysfunction in women: A review of population-based studies. *Journal of Sexual Medicine, 2,* 317–330.

Heavey, C., Christensen, A., & Malamuth, N. (1995). The longitudinal impact of demand and withdrawal during marital conflict. *Journal of Consulting and Clinical Psychology, 63,* 797–801.

Heiman, J. R. (2007). Orgasmic disorders in women. In S. R. Leiblum (Ed.), *Principles and practice of sex therapy* (4th ed., pp. 84–123). New York: Guilford Press.

Herbenick, D., Reece, M., Sanders, S., Dodge, B., Ghassemi, A., & Fortenberry, J. D. (2009). Prevalence and characteristics of vibrator use by women in the United States: Results from a nationally representative study. *Journal of Sexual Medicine, 6*, 1857–1866.

Herbenick, D., Schick, V., Reece, M., Sanders, S., Dodge, B., & Fortenberry, J. D. (2011). The Female Genital Self-Image Scale (FGSIS): Results from a nationally representative probability sample of women in the United States. *Journal of Sexual Medicine, 8*, 158–166.

Hudson, W. W., Harrison, D. F., & Crossup, P. C. (1981). A short form scale to measure sexual discord in dyadic relationships. *Journal of Sex Research, 17*, 157–174.

Hurlbert, D. F. (1993). A comparative study using orgasm consistency training in the treatment of women reporting hypoactive sexual desire. *Journal of Sex and Marital Therapy, 19*, 41–55.

IsHak, W. W., Bokarious, A., Jeffrey, J. K., Davis, M. C., & Bakhta, Y. (2010). Disorders of orgasm in women: A literature review of etiology and current treatments. *Journal of Sexual Medicine, 7*, 3254–3268.

Janssen, E., McBride, K. R., Yarber, W., Hill, B. J., & Butler, S. M. (2008). Factors that influence sexual arousal in men: A focus group study. *Archives of Sexual Behavior, 37*, 252–265.

Jiann, B. P., Su, C. C., Yu, C. C., Wu, T. T., & Huang, J.-K. (2009). Risk factors for individual domains of female sexual function. *Journal of Sexual Medicine, 6*, 3364–75.

Justman. S. (2011). From medicine to psychotherapy: The placebo effect. *History of the Human Sciences, 24*, 95–107.

Kaplan, H. S. (1974). *The new sex therapy.* New York: Brunner/Mazel.

Kaplan, H. S. (1977). Hypoactive sexual desire. *Journal of Sex and Marital Therapy, 3*, 3–9.

Katz, R. C., Gipson, M. T., Kearl, A., & Kriskovich, M. (1989). Assessing sexual aversion in college students: The Sexual Aversion Scale. *Journal of Sex and Marital Therapy, 15*, 135–140.

Kazdin, A. E. (2008). Evidence-based treatment and practice: New opportunities to bridge clinical research and practice, enhance the knowledge base, and improve patient care. *American Psychologist, 63*, 146–159.

Kennedy, S. H., Dickens, S. E., Eisfeld, B. S., & Bagby, M. (1999). Sexual dysfunction before antidepressant therapy for major depression. *Journal of Affective Disorders, 56*, 201–208.

Klaassen, M., & ter Kuile, M. M. (2009). Development and initial validation of the Vaginal Penetration Cognition Questionnaire (VPCQ) in a sample of women with vaginismus and dyspareunia. *Journal of Sexual Medicine, 6*, 1617–1627.

Lai, Y, & Hynie, M. (2011). A tale of two standards: An examination of young adults' endorsement of gendered and ageist sexual double standards. *Sex Roles, 64*, 360–371.

Landry, T., Bergeron, S., Dupuis, M.-J., & Desrochers, G. (2008). The treatment of provoked vestibulodynia: A critical review. *Clinical Journal of Pain, 24*, 155–171.

Latthe, P., Mignini, L., Gray, R., Hills, R., & Khan, K. (2006). Factors predisposing women to chronic pelvic pain: A systematic review. *British Medical Journal, 332*, 749–755.

Laumann, E. O., Gagnon, J. H., Michael, R. T., & Michaels, S. (1994). *The social organization of sexuality: Sexual practices in the United States.* Chicago, IL: University of Chicago Press.

Laumann, E. O., Nicolosi, A., Glasser, D. B., Paik, A., Gingell, C., Moreira, E., ... Wang, T. (2005). Sexual problems among women and men aged 40–80 years: Prevalence and correlates identified by the Global Study of Sexual Attitudes and Behaviors. *International Journal of Impotence Research, 17*, 39–57.

Laumann, E. O., Paik, A., & Rosen, R. C. (1999). Sexual dysfunction in the United States: Prevalence and predictors. *Journal of the American Medical Association, 281*, 537–544.

Leiblum, S. R., Koochaki, P. E., Rodenberg, C. A., Barton, I. P., & Rosen, R. C. (2006). Hypoactive sexual desire disorder in postmenopausal women: US results from the Women's International Study of Health and Sexuality (WISHeS). *Menopause, 13*, 46–56.

Leonard, L. M., & Follette, V. M. (2002). Sexual functioning in women reporting a history of child sexual abuse: Review of the empirical literature and clinical implications. *Annual Review of Sex Research, 13,* 346–388.

Levin, R. J. (2004). Measuring female genital function: A research essential but still a clinical luxury? *Sexual and Relationship Therapy, 19,* 191–200.

Lewis, R. W., Fugl-Meyer, K. S., Corona, G., Hayes, R. D., Laumann, E. O., Rellini, A., & Segraves, T. (2010). Definitions/epidemiology/risk factors for sexual dysfunction. *Journal of Sexual Medicine, 7,* 1598–1607.

Lief, H. I. (1977). Inhibited sexual desire. *Medical Aspects of Human Sexuality, 7,* 94–95.

LoPiccolo, J., & Steger, J.C. (1974). The Sexual Interaction Inventory: A new instrument for assessment of sexual dysfunction. *Archives of Sexual Behavior, 3,* 585–595.

Lykins, A. D., Meana, M., & Minimi, J. (2011). Visual attention to erotic images in women reporting pain with intercourse. *Journal of Sex Research, 48,* 43–52.

MacPhee, D. C., Johnson, S. M., & van der Veer, M. M. C. (1995). Low sexual desire in women: The effects of marital therapy. *Journal of Sex and Marital Therapy, 21,* 159–182.

Mah, K., & Binik, Y. M. (2001). The nature of the human orgasm. A critical review of major trends. *Clinical Psychology Review, 21,* 823–856.

Masters, W. H., & Johnson, V. E. (1970). *Human sexual inadequacy.* London: Little, Brown.

McCarthy, B. W. (1993). Relapse prevention strategies and techniques in sex therapy. *Journal of Sex and Marital Therapy, 19,* 142–146.

McCormick, N. (2010). Sexual scripts: Social and therapeutic implications. *Sexual and Relationship Therapy, 25,* 96–120.

McCoy, N., L., & Matyas, J. R. (1998). McCoy Female Sexuality Questionnaire. In C. M. Davis, W. L. Yarber, R. Bauserman, G. Schreer, & S. L. Davis (Eds.), *Handbook of sexuality related measures* (pp. 249–251). Thousand Oaks, CA: Sage.

Meana, M. (2010). Elucidating women's (hetero)sexual desire: Definitional challenges and content expansion. *Journal of Sex Research, 47,* 104–122.

Meana, M., Binik, Y. M., Khalife, S., & Cohen, D. (1997a). Dyspareunia: Sexual dysfunction or pain syndrome? *Journal of Nervous and Mental Disease, 185,* 561–569.

Meana, M., Binik, Y. M., Khalife, S., & Cohen, D. (1997b). Biopsychosocial profile of women with dyspareunia. *Obstetrics & Gynecology, 90,* 583–589.

Meana, M., Binik, Y. M., Khalife, S., & Cohen, D. (1998). Affect and marital adjustment in women's rating of dyspareunic pain. *Canadian Journal of Psychiatry, 43, 381–385.*

Meana, M., Binik, Y. M., Khalife, S., & Cohen, D. (1999). Psychosocial correlates of pain attributions in women with dyspareunia. *Psychosomatics, 40,* 497–502.

Meana, M., Binik, Y. M., & Thaler, L. (2008). Sexual dysfunction. In J. Hunsley & E. Mash (Eds.), *A guide to assessments that work* (pp. 464–487). New York: Oxford University Press.

Meana, M., & Lykins, A. D. (2009). Negative affect and somatically focused anxiety in young women reporting pain with intercourse. *Journal of Sex Research, 46,* 80–88.

Meana, M., & Nunnink, S. E. (2006). Gender differences in the content of cognitive distraction during sex. *Journal of Sex Research, 43,* 59–67.

Melzack, R. (1975). The McGill Pain Questionnaire: Major properties and scoring methods. *Pain, 1,* 277–299.

Mercer, C. H., Fenton, K. A., Johnson, A. M., Wellings, K., Macdowell, W., McManus, S., ... Erens, B. (2003). Sexual function problems and help seeking behaviour in Britain: National probability samples survey. *British Medical Journal, 327,* 426–427.

Meston, C. M., & Bradford, A. (2007). Autonomic nervous system influences: The role of the sympathetic nervous system in female sexual arousal. In E. Janssen (Ed.), *The psychophysiology of sex* (pp. 66–82). Bloomington, IN: Indiana University Press.

Meston, C. M., & Heiman, J. R. (2000). Sexual abuse and sexual function: An examination of sexually relevant cognitive processes. *Journal of Consulting and Clinical Psychology, 68,* 399–406.

Meston, C. M., Hull, E., Levin, R. J., & Sipski, M. (2004). Disorders of orgasm in women. *Journal of Sexual Medicine, 1,* 66–68.

Meston, C. M., & Trapnell, P. (2005). Development and validation of a five-factor sexual satisfaction and distress scale for women: The Sexual Satisfaction Scale for women. *Journal of Sexual Medicine, 2,* 66–81.

Milhausen, R. R., Graham, C. A., Sanders, S. A., Yarber, W. L., & Maitland, S. B. (2010). Validation of the Sex Excitation/Sex Inhibition Inventory for women and men. *Archives of Sexual Behavior, 39,* 1091–1104.

Miller, W. R., & Rollnick, S. (1991). *Motivational interviewing.* London: Guilford Press.

Moser, C. (2009). Autogynephilia in women. *Journal of Homosexuality, 56,* 539–547.

Muehlenhard, C. L., & Shippee, S. K. (2010). Men's and women's reports of pretending orgasm. *Journal of Sex Research, 47,* 552–567.

Nicholls, L. (2008). Putting the New View classification scheme to an empirical test. *Feminism and Psychology, 18,* 515–526.

Nichols, M., & Shernoff, M. (2007). Therapy with sexual minorities. In S. R. Leiblum (Ed.), *Principles and practice of sex therapy* (4th ed., pp. 379–415). New York: Guilford Press.

Nicolson, P., & Burr, J. (2003). What is 'normal' about women's (hetero)sexual desire and orgasm? A report of an in-depth interview study. *Social Science and Medicine, 57,* 1735–1745.

Nobre, P. J., & Pinto-Gouveia, J. (2006). Emotions during sexual activity: Differences between sexually functional and dysfunctional men and women. *Archives of Sexual Behavior, 35,* 491–499.

Nobre, P. J., & Pinto-Gouveia, J. (2008). Cognitions, emotions, and sexual response: Analysis of the relationship among automatic thoughts, emotional responses, and sexual arousal. *Archives of Sexual Behavior, 37,* 652–661.

Oberg, K., Fugl-Meyer, A. R., & Fugl-Meyer, K. S. (2004). On categorization and quantification of women's sexual dysfunctions: An epidemiological approach. *International Journal of Impotence Research, 16,* 261–269.

Oppenheimer, C. (2002). Sexuality in old age. In R. Jacoby & C. Oppenheimer (Eds.), *Psychiatry in the elderly* (pp. 37–60). Oxford: Oxford University Press.

Payne, K., Binik, Y. M., Amsel, R., & Khalife, S. (2005). When sex hurts, anxiety and fear orient attention towards pain. *European Journal of Pain, 9,* 427–36.

Perelman, M. A. (2009). Sexual Tipping Point®: A mind/body model for sexual medicine. *Journal of Sexual Medicine, 6,* 629–632.

Petersen, C. M, Giraldi, A., Lundvall, L., & Kristensen, E. (2009). Botulinum toxin type A: A novel treatment for provoked vestibulodynia? Results from a randomized, placebo controlled, double blinded study. *Journal of Sexual Medicine, 6,* 2523–2537.

Prochaska, J. O., & Prochaska, J. M. (1999). Why don't continents move? Why don't people change? *Journal of Psychotherapy Integration, 9,* 83–102.

Pukall, C. F., Binik, Y. M., & Khalife, S. (2004). A new instrument for pain assessment in vulvar vestibulitis syndrome. *Journal of Sex and Marital Therapy, 30,* 69–78.

Pukall, C. F., Strigo, I. A., Binik, Y. M., Amsel, R., Khalife, S., & Bushnell, M. C. (2005). Neural correlates of painful genital touch in women with vulvar vestibulitis. *Pain, 115,* 118–127.

Quirk, F. H., Heiman, J. R., Rosen, R. C., Laan, E., Smith, M. D., & Boolell, M. (2002). Development of a sexual function questionnaire for clinical trials of female sexual dysfunction. *Journal of Women's Health and Gender-Based Medicine, 11,* 277–289.

Reissing, E., Binik, Y. M., Khalife, S., Cohen, D., & Amsel, R. (2003). Etiological correlates of vaginismus: Sexual and physical abuse, sexual knowledge, sexual self-schema, and relationship adjustment. *Journal of Sex and Marital Therapy, 29,* 47–59.

Reissing, E., Binik, Y. M., Khalife, S., Cohen, D., & Amsel, R. (2004). Vaginal spasm, pain and behavior: An empirical investigation of vaginismus. *Archives of Sexual Behavior, 33,* 5–17.

Reissing, E., Brown, C., Lord, M. J., Binik, Y. M., & Khalife, S. (2005). Pelvic floor muscle functioning in women with vulvar vestibulitis syndrome. *Journal of Psychosomatic Obstetrics and Gynecology, 26,* 107–113.

Rellini, A. H., & Meston, C. M. (2006). Psychophysiological sexual arousal in women with a history of child sexual abuse. *Journal of Sex and Marital Therapy, 32,* 5–22.

Rosen, R., Brown, C., Heiman, J. Leiblum, S., Meston, C., Shabsigh, R., ... D'Agostino, R., Jr. (2000). The Female Sexual Function Index (FSFI): A multidimensional self-report instrument for the assessment of female sexual function. *Journal of Sex and Marital Therapy, 26,* 191–208.

Rosen, R. C., Cappelleri, J. C., & Gendrano, N., III. (2002). The international index of erectile function (IIEF): A state-of-the-science review. *International Journal of Impotence Research, 14,* 226–244.

Rosen, R. C., Cappelleri, J. C., Smith, M. D., Lipsky, J., & Pena, B. M. (1999). Development and evaluation of an abridged, 5-item version of the international index of erectile function (IIEF-5) as a diagnostic tool for erectile dysfunction. *International Journal of Impotence Research, 11,* 319–326.

Rosen, R. C., Catania, J., Pollack, L., Althof, S., O'Leary, M., & Seftel, A. D. (2004). Male Sexual Health Questionnaire (MSHQ): Scale development and psychometric validation. *Urology, 64,* 777–782.

Rosen, R. C., Lane, R. M., & Menza, M. (1999). Effects of SSRI's on sexual function: A critical review. *Journal of Clinical Psychopharmacology, 19,* 67–85.

Rosen, R. C., Lobo, R.A., Block, B.A., Ynag, H.-M., & Zipfel, L. M. (2004). Menopausal Sexual Interest Questionnaire (MSIQ): A unidimensional scale for the assessment of sexual interest in postmenopausal women. *Journal of Sex and Marital Therapy, 30,* 235–250.

Rosenbaum, T. Y., & Owens, A. (2008). The role of pelvic floor physical therapy in the treatment of pelvic and genital pain-related sexual dysfunction. *Journal of Sexual Medicine, 5,* 513–523.

Rust, J., & Golombok, S. (1986). The GRISS: A psychometric instrument for the assessment of sexual dysfunction. *Archives of Sexual Behavior, 15,* 157–165.

Schnarch, D. M. (2003). *Resurrecting sex: Solving sexual problems and revolutionizing your relationship.* New York: Harper Paperbacks.

Segraves, K. B. & Segraves, R. T. (1991). Hypoactive sexual desire disorder: Prevalence and comorbidity in 906 subjects. *Journal of Sex and Marital Therapy, 17,* 55–58.

Shifren, J. L., Monz, B. U., Russo, P. A., Segreti, A., & Johannes, C. B. (2008). Sexual problems and distress in United States women. *Obstetrics and Gynecology, 112,* 970–978.

Sills, T., Wunderlich, G., Pyke, R., Segraves, R. T., Leiblum, S., Clayton, A., ... Evans, K. (2005). The Sexual Interest and Desire Inventory – Female (SIDI-F): Item response analyses of data from women diagnosed with hypoactive sexual desire disorder. *Journal of Sexual Medicine, 2,* 801–818.

Sims, K. E., & Meana, M. (2010). Why did passion wane? A qualitative study of married women's attributions for declines in sexual desire. *Journal of Sex and Marital Therapy, 36,* 360–380.

Spanier, G. B. (1976). Measuring dyadic adjustment: New scales for assessing the quality of marriage and similar dyads. *Journal of Marriage and Family, 38,* 15–28.

Spector, I. P., Carey, M. P., & Steinberg, L. (1996). The Sexual Desire Inventory: Development, factor structure, and evidence of reliability. *Journal of Sex and Marital Therapy, 22,* 175– 190.

Sprecher, S., & Cate, R. M. (2004). Sexual satisfaction and sexual expression as predictors of relationship satisfaction and stability. In J. Harvey, A. Wenzel, & S. Sprecher (Eds.), *Handbook of sexuality in close relationships* (pp. 235–256). Mahwah, NJ: Erlbaum.

Sullivan, M. J. L., Bishop, S. R., & Pivik, J. (1995). The Pain Catastrophizing Scale: Development and validation. *Psychological Assessment, 7,* 524–532.

Sullivan, M. J. L., Lynch, M. E., & Clark, A. J. (2005). Dimensions of catastrophic thinking associated with pain experience and disability in patients with neuropathic pain conditions. *Pain, 113,* 310–315.

Taylor, J. F., Rosen, R. C., & Leiblum, S. R. (1994). Self-report assessment of female sexual function: Psychometric evaluation of the Brief Index of Sexual Functioning for Women. *Archives of Sexual Behavior, 23,* 627–643.

ter Kuile, M. M., Both, S., van Lankveld, J. D. M. (2010). Cognitive behavioral therapy for sexual dysfunctions in women. *Psychiatric Clinics in North America, 33,* 595–610.

Tiefer, L. (2001). A new view of women's sexual problems: Why new? Why now? *Journal of Sex Research, 38,* 89–96.

Tolman, D. L. (2002). Dilemmas of desire: Teenage girls talk about sexuality. Cambridge, MA: Harvard University Press.

Trapnell, P. D., Meston, C. M., & Gorzalka, B. B. (1997). Spectatoring and the relationship between body image and sexual experience: Self-focus or self-valence? *Journal of Sex Research, 34,* 267–278.

Trudel, G., Marchand, A., Ravart, M., Aubin, S, Turgeon, L., & Fortier, P. (2001). The effect of a cognitive behavioral treatment program on hypoactive sexual desire in women. *Sexual and Relationship Therapy, 16,* 145–164.

Tuiten, A., Laan, E., Panhuysen, G., Everaerd, W., de Haan, F., Koppeschaar, H., & Vroon, P. (1996). Discrepancies between genital responses and subjective sexual function during testosterone substitution in women with hypothalamic amenorrhea. *Psychosomatic Medicine, 58,* 234–241.

van Lankveld, J. (2008). Problems with sexual interest and desire. In D. L. Rowland & L. Incrocci (Eds.), *Handbook of sexual and gender identity disorders* (pp. 154–187). Hoboken, NJ: Wiley.

van Lankveld, J. (2009). Self-help therapies for sexual dysfunction. *Journal of Sex Research, 46,* 143–155.

Weeks, G. R. & Cross, C. (2004). The intersystem model of psychotherapy: An integrative systems approach. *Guidance and Counseling, 19,* 57–64.

Weeks, G. R, & Gambescia, N. (2009). A systemic approach to sensate focus. In K. M. Hertlein, G. R. Weeks, & N. Gambescia (Eds.), *Systemic sex therapy*. New York: Routledge.

West, S. L., D'Aloisio, A. A., Agans, R. P., Kalsbeek, W. D., Borisov, N. N., & Thorp, J. M. (2008). Prevalence of low desire and hypoactive sexual desire disorder in a nationally representative sample of U.S. women. *Archives of Internal Medicine, 168,* 1441–1449.

Wiederman, M. W. (2000). Women's body image self-consciousness during physical intimacy with a partner. *Journal of Sex Research, 37,* 60–68.

Wierman, M. E., Nappi, R. E., Avis, N., Davis, S. R., Labrie, F., Rosner, W., & Shifren, J. L. (2010). Endocrine aspects of women's sexual function. *Journal of Sexual Medicine, 7,* 561–585.

Witting, K., Santtila, P., Rijsdijk, F., Varjonen, M., Jern, P., Johansson, A., . . . Sandnabba, N. K. (2009). Correlated genetic and non-shared environmental influences account for the comorbidity between female sexual dysfunctions. *Psychological Medicine, 39,* 115–127.

Working Group on a New View of Women's Sexual Problems. (2000). *The New View Manifesto: A new view of women's sexual problems.* Retrieved http://www.fsd-alert.org

World Health Organization. (1992). *Manual of the international statistical classification of diseases and related health problems* (10th ed.). Geneva: Author.

8

Appendix: Tools and Resources

Appendix 1: Useful Addresses
Appendix 2: Clinical Interview: Questions Related to Diagnostic Criteria and
Specifiers
Appendix 3: Clinical Interview: Assessment of Client/Partner History and
Possible Dimensional Specifiers

Appendix 1

Useful Addresses

Clinically-Oriented Sexuality Associations
These associations provide continuing education related to the treatment of sexual problems.

American Association for Sex Educators, Counselors and Therapists (AASECT)
PO Box 1960
Ashland, Virginia 23005-1960
USA
Tel. +1 804 752-0026
Web: http://www.aasect.org

International Society for the Study of Women's Sexual Health (ISSWSH)
Two Woodfield Lake
1100 E. Woodfield Rd., Suite 520
Schaumburg, IL 60173
USA
Tel. +1 847 517-7225
Web: http://www.isswsh.org

Society for Sex Therapy and Research (SSTAR)
6311 W. Gross Point Road
Niles, Illinois 60714
USA
Tel. +1 847 647-8832
Web: http://www.sstarnet.org

Professional Associations for Allied Health Professionals
The following associations can be useful for specialized referrals to gynecologists, physical therapists, or vulvar pain specialists. They also have good resources and information for clients.

American College of Obstetrics & Gynecology (ACOG)
409 12th Street SW
PO Box 96920
Washington, DC 20090-6920
USA
Tel. +1 202 638-5577
Web: http://www.acog.org

American Association of Physical Therapists (APTA)
1111 North Fairfax Street
Alexandria, Virginia 22314-1488
USA
Tel. +1 703 684-2782
Web: http://www.apta.org

National Vulvodynia Association (NVA)
PO Box 4491
Silver Spring, MD 20914-4491
USA
Tel. +1 301 299-0775
Web: http://www.nva.org

North American Menopause Society (NAMS)
PO Box 94527
Cleveland, Ohio 44101
Tel. +1 440 442-7550
Web: http://www.menopause.org

Online Sources for the Purchase of Vaginal Dilators
http://www.vaginismus.com
http://www.pureromance.com
http://www.soulsourceenterprises.com
http://www.a-woman's-touch.com

Videos and Other Media for Clients
Sinclair Intimacy Institute (*DVDs and videos related to sexual instruction and enhancement*)
Web: http://www.bettersex.com

Betty Dodson with Carlin Ross (*information, media, and products related to women's sexuality*)
Web: http://www.dodsonandross.com

Kinsey Confidential (*web-based Q&A and media on sexual topics*)
Web: http://www.kinseyconfidential.org

Online Sex Toy Boutiques
A Woman's Touch
http://www.a-woman's-touch.com

Babeland
http://www.babeland.com

Good Vibrations
http://www.goodvibes.com

My Pleasure
http://www.mypleasure.com

Tulip
http://www.mytulip.com

Appendix 2

Clinical Interview: Questions Related to Diagnostic Criteria and Specifiers

Criteria/Specifiers	Questions
Desire/Aversion/Arousal	• How often are you interested in sexual activity (partnered or solitary masturbation)? • How often do you have erotic thoughts or fantasies? • How often do you initiate sex? • How often are you responsive to sex when initiated by your partner? • How often do you have feelings of anxiety, fear, or disgust when you think of or are engaged in sex? • How often do you feel "turned on" or experience pleasure once sexual activity has started? • How often do you feel that your genitals and body fail to respond sufficiently to sexual stimulation? (e.g., insufficient sustained lubrication, lack of tingling, swelling, pulsing and/or other sensation that used to accompany arousal)
Orgasm	• How often do your reach orgasm with partnered sex? with masturbation? • How often are orgasms difficult to reach? • How often do you find that the intensity of the orgasm is weak?
Dyspareunia/Vaginismus	• How often are you unable to have sexual intercourse (vaginal penetration) when you try? • How often do you have pain during sexual intercourse? • How often do you experience fear of penetration or pain when you try to have intercourse? • How often do you feel that muscles in your genital area tense up when you try to or have intercourse?
Distress	• How distressing is this problem to you? How does it make you feel? What is your general reaction to it? • Has this problem resulted in interpersonal difficulty for you? Please describe in what ways. • How satisfied are you with your sexual life?
Onset	• Has the problem been lifelong or did it start at some later point? • Was there anything going on in your life or your body at the time that the problems started that you think might be related to onset? Since the problem started, has it gotten worse, stayed the same, or improved?
Context	• Does the problem occur in all situations or does it depend on certain conditions? (e.g., a specific partner, his/her mood, life circumstances, etc.) • Are there conditions in your life that improve it or make it worse?
Etiology	• Do you have any theories or ideas about what has brought about or caused this problem? • Do you have any theories or ideas about factors in your life that are interfering with a possible resolution to the problem? • To what extent do you think this is a psychological problem that rests within you? • To what extent do you think this is a relational problem reflecting problems in your relationship? • To what extent do you think this is a medical/physical problem?

From: M. Meana: *Sexual Dysfunction in Women*   © 2012 Hogrefe Publishing

Appendix 3

Clinical Interview: Assessment of Client/Partner History and Possible Dimensional Specifiers

Sexual Dysfunction Treatment History
Health professional delivered prior treatment attempts for the problem and their outcome
Informal personal attempts to treat/manage the problem and their outcome

Sexual and Relationship History
First sexual experiences
Family of origin attitudes about sex
Client attitudes/expectations about sex
Sexual self-concept
Sexual self-efficacy
Nature of sexual relationships in the past (casual and committed)
Sexual trauma

Current Relationship
Satisfaction with nonsexual aspects of the relationship (e.g., communication, affection)
Satisfaction with partner sexual skill
Physical attraction to partner
Discrepancies in desire
Partner causal attributions for the problem
Partner reactions to the problem
Partner sexual dysfunction
Partner general health

Psychological Well-Being
Mood and emotional regulation
Cognitive style (ruminative? hypervigilant? inattentive?)
Body image
History of mental health problems
Life satisfaction

Current Life Circumstances
Marital status
Children (how many? how old?)
Employment (fulfilling?)
Financial security
Situational stressors

Medical History (Past and Current)
Medical conditions (see Table 4)
Medications (see Table 4)
Treatments and surgeries (see Table 4)
Chronic pain
Lifestyle factors (e.g., body mass index, smoking, substance use)

Cultural
Ethnocultural or religious beliefs/values regarding sexuality
Adherence/conflict with these beliefs/values

From: M. Meana: *Sexual Dysfunction in Women* © 2012 Hogrefe Publishing